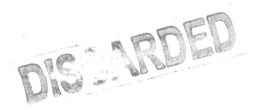

GOING HIGHER

GOING HIGHER

The Story of Man and Altitude
Revised Edition

Charles S. Houston, M.D.

Illustrations by Gary Nelson

LITTLE, BROWN AND COMPANY

Boston   Toronto

THIRD EDITION, REVISED

Library of Congress Cataloging-in-Publication Data

Houston, Charles S.
  Going higher.

  Bibliography: p.
  Includes index.
  1. Mountaineering — Physiological aspects. 2. Altitude, In-
fluence of. I. Title. [DNLM: 1. Adaptation, Physiological. 2.
Altitude. 3. Mountaineering. WD 710 H843g]
RC1220.M6H68   1987   616.9′893   86-20809
ISBN 0-316-37445-8
ISBN 0-316-37446-6 (pbk.)

RRD VA

Published simultaneously in Canada
by Little, Brown & Company (Canada) Limited

PRINTED IN THE UNITED STATES OF AMERICA

CONTENTS

List of Illustrations   vii

Preface   Why This Book?   ix

Chapter One   Men and Mountains   3

Chapter Two   Toward Understanding the Physical Universe   16

Chapter Three   Exploration of the Heavens   46

Chapter Four   Moving Air: Respiration   66

Chapter Five   Moving Blood: Circulation   82

Chapter Six   Transporting Oxygen: Hemoglobin   91

Chapter Seven   Using Oxygen: The Cell   105

Chapter Eight   Altitude Illness   122

Chapter Nine   Acute Mountain Sickness (AMS)   134

Chapter Ten   High-Altitude Pulmonary Edema (HAPE)   146

Chapter Eleven   High-Altitude Cerebral Edema (HACE)   169

Chapter Twelve   Other Altitude Problems   181

Chapter Thirteen   Acclimatization   201

Chapter Fourteen   Women at Altitude   230

Chapter Fifteen   On the Summit   241

Altitude and Barometric Pressure   254

People in Altitude Physiology 257
Glossary 271
Bibliography 277
  Books 278
  Papers 286
Index 318

ILLUSTRATIONS

Figure   Page
1   Acosta's Map of Pariacaca   13
2   The First "Barometer"   18–19
3   Guericke Demonstrates the Weight of the
    Atmosphere   22
4   Perier Prepares to Climb the Puy du Dôme   24
5   Robert Hooke's "Decompression Chamber"   26–27
6   Life in a Vacuum: The Benefits of Oxygen   29
7   Lavoisier in His Laboratory   36
8   There Were (Allegedly) Dragons on the Mountains   40
9   De Saussure on Mont Blanc: The First Scientist-
    Climber   42
10 Would This "Airship" Really Fly?   49
11 The First Free Balloon Flight — 1783   52
12 Balloons Created Special Problems   53
13 Paul Bert's Decompression Chamber   58
14 The Oxygen Cascade   70–71
15 Respiration: How Air Enters and Leaves the Lungs   72
16 The Lung Capillaries and Alveoli   74–75
17 Defining Ventilation   79
18 Changes in Alveolar Gases at Altitude   80
19 Circulation: How Blood Moves Throughout
    the Body   86–87
20 Oxygen Transport: Red Blood Cells and
    Hemoglobin   93

21 The Oxy-Hemoglobin Dissociation Curve   96–97
22 The Kidneys   102
23 Robert Hooke's Microscope   107
24 The Cell: Its Membrane and Mitochondria   110
25 The Cell's Metabolism and Energy
    Production   114–115
26 The Sodium Pump   118–119
27 Physical and Mental Changes During Rapid Ascent 123
28 Normal and Fluid-filled Alveoli   148
29 A Typical Case of High-Altitude Pulmonary Edema 151
30 Various Forms of High-Altitude Pulmonary
    Edema   154–155
31 The Brain in Its Rigid Box   172
32 Too Many Red Blood Cells May Be
    Disadvantageous   183
33 The Retina and Its Blood Vessels at Sea Level
    and at Altitude   186
34 Haldane and Friends on Pikes Peak in 1911   206
35 The Silver Hut — Near Everest in 1961   210
36 "Logan High" — the Arctic Institute's Altitude
    Laboratory   213
37 Early Women Climbers   232–233
38 Operation Everest, 1946   244
39 Operation Everest II, 1985   247

WHY THIS BOOK?

FIRST MOUNTAINEERING and later high-altitude physiology have been major parts of my life, and I have long wanted to write a book about the two. From 1975 to 1983 I stumbled through many drafts, only to have the manuscript rejected by a dozen publishers: "Too long," "Too technical," "Not scientific enough," they said — or, most often, "Who will read it?" In short: failure. So I took my courage in both hands and published the book myself, fortunately finding the right designer (Craig Dicken at Battery Graphics), a splendid artist (Gary Nelson), and a sympathetic printer (Allan Schillhammer at Queen City Printers) in Burlington. After two editions sold out, Little, Brown invited me to do a new and expanded edition.

But why bother? High altitude and the problems it can cause affect only a few venturesome skiers and climbers. Compared to death by automobiles, alcohol and drugs, or the looming Armageddon, altitude illness is trivial. But more and more people are going to the mountains, and too many are getting sick at altitudes thought to be innocuous. Some are dying — unnecessarily. Research in high altitude has become intense, and there is growing interest in the similarities and differences between healthy climbers on high mountains and sick people at sea level. The more we look, the more we realize how little we really know and how much we still have to learn.

People are also becoming more curious about how their bodies work and how to stay healthy. Masses run, ski, trek, lift weights, join health clubs, and to their surprise find that they really do feel better and soon come to enjoy the workouts. There's been a great surge of literature about wellness and about science, particularly the biological sciences. Television allows millions to peer into the most intimate crevices of living organisms and to look at the immensity of space, though we can't comprehend either. We watch an ovum mature to a newborn babe; we can "make" new organisms by tinkering with the genetic code. Every day seems to bring new knowledge — but does understanding come with it?

At the same time, as science advances, it is accompanied by a cloud of confusion and contradiction and by difficult ethical and moral choices. Risks and benefits are harder to evaluate. If we can't understand science, how can we hope to use it appropriately?

It seems to me that part of a physician's obligation is to help people, sick or well, to better understand these choices and these issues, and to do so we all need to understand how our bodies function. Better health depends on better understanding. Wellness is more than the absence of disease.

So I wrote this book to describe how we came to learn what we know today, trying to explain how man lives in this wonder-filled world, and how we may avoid a few of the hazards. I hoped to express some of the excitement of exploration and the satisfaction of discovery. I chose to aim for clarity at the expense of completeness, trying to be as accurate as necessary but as simple as possible. I strove for a book that would be enjoyable as well as informative and useful, a book which would interest doctors and nonscientists, climbers, balloonists, trekkers, skiers — and those who might never go above sea level. I was encouraged in this thought when the woman who set the type for the first edition told me how much the book had helped her to understand her husband's death from lung cancer.

Since my first edition, the published work on hypoxia has increased enormously. Consequently I have more than doubled the bibliography for those who want more detailed scientific data than I thought appropriate to include in the text. Even so, the bibliography is very far from complete — it is but a door through which those interested can enter the great world of literature about high altitude.

Few people write without help. I am deeply indebted to the many who told me about interesting cases and to others who pointed out my errors of omission or commission. To Galen Rowell I owe special thanks for the magnificent selection of photographs he sent me from which to choose for the cover, and for the elegance with which he expresses his mountaineering philosophy and ethics. Doctors David Schlim, Herbert Hultgren, Rob Schoene, and Drummond Rennie have helped more in the scientific aspects than they may realize. Many people I do not know encouraged me. Chris Coffin and Peggy Freudenthal at Little, Brown showed me that some professional publishers can be user-friendly. Craig Dicken has as always been a patient and imaginative cover designer. It's been a most rewarding venture which my wife and I have shared, and she should be my co-author.

Burlington, Vermont
October 1986

GOING HIGHER

Whatever you can do,
    Or think you can, begin it.
Boldness has power, and genius,
    And magic in it.

— *Johann Wolfgang von Goethe*

Chapter One

MEN AND MOUNTAINS

A PECULIARLY HUMAN initiative is testing limits, seeking new frontiers to breach in exploration or science or sport. We are restless seekers, quickly tiring of the familiar, hopeful that more or new will be better. We have been miles deep into the earth and to the bottom of the seas and to the tops of the highest mountains. Finally we are venturing into space, to which there is no limit, no boundary to pass.

Oceans, deserts, polar wastes, quiet forests, vast plains, and icy mountains all draw pilgrims of various purpose. Some come humbly, others to conquer, some for refreshment, others to learn. Dreams of flying or of being high above the ordinary world have captured human imagination throughout the centuries. Reaching a high place is an exciting challenge, a visible, tangible goal, a set task accomplished, something ventured, something won. Mountains are awesome, magnificent or fearsome, undeniable, immovable — but obstacles that can be overcome. The 121st Psalm is inspiring: "I will lift up mine eyes unto the hills, from whence cometh my help." Moses went to the summit to bring down the word of God. Isaiah urged, "Get thee up into the high mountains." William Blake's often-quoted verse is more pragmatic: "Great things are done when men and mountains meet. . . ."

Climbing offers many things to many people but entails risks in addition to its rewards. As more and more people go to the higher mountains, these dangers are taking an increasing toll, which need not be paid if people are mindful of the dangers and how they can be minimized. High altitude can affect anyone — even the most experienced climber — who is unwary or uninformed. Cold and lack of oxygen go hand in hand on high mountains, and both can cripple or kill. Altitude sickness may be fatal because, like other mammals, we are completely dependent on oxygen, and as altitude increases, the available oxygen decreases. Understanding why we need and how we obtain oxygen and how we adjust to oxygen lack is the surest way to stay well on high mountains.

A healthy thirty-eight-year-old man drove from his home at 5,200 feet to 9,600 feet for a weekend of tennis. On Saturday he was somewhat short of breath but kept up with his peers. That night his shortness of breath grew worse and he coughed a great deal. On Sunday he was able to play only briefly before the shortness of breath alarmed him so much that he drove home, where he still was short of breath. On Monday morning, coughing up frothy bloody sputum, he was admitted to a hospital where a diagnosis of high-altitude pulmonary edema was made. He recovered within twenty-four hours.

A middle-aged dentist reached 9,600 feet six hours after leaving home at sea level. That evening he felt as though he had flu and developed slight fever, nausea, and diarrhea. Next morning he was very weak and short of breath and was coughing severely. He was taken down to 8,000 feet but did not improve. Next day he grew worse despite antibiotics prescribed by telephone. He became irrational during the night and died at dawn about sixty hours after leaving sea level. Postmortem X ray showed extensive pulmonary edema, but a complication (Legionnaire's Disease) was suspected though not provable.

A young teacher drove from sea level to 8,400 feet in forty-eight hours and spent two days there. During the next four days he and his friends, carrying fifty-pound packs, skied slowly up to 10,500 feet, although he soon developed a headache, which grew worse each day. On the fourth day he had trouble breathing and could barely travel. That night his companions noticed a rattling sound when he breathed, and he was barely conscious. When a rescue helicopter arrived on the sixth morning he was comatose and on arrival at a hospital was found to have severe pulmonary edema (fluid in both lungs), hemorrhages in both eyes, and evidence of brain damage. He regained consciousness slowly and was discharged after five days. Since this incident he has several times climbed slowly to 11,000 feet without difficulty.

A healthy man walked from 5,000 to 16,000 feet in five days. There he became very tired, developed a severe headache, and had difficulty keeping his balance. He became increasingly short of breath. He descended to 14,000 feet with difficulty and rested for three days, but his condition deteriorated and he was air-lifted to a hospital where he remained for eleven days under intensive treatment. He had brain and pulmonary edema due to altitude, and hemorrhages in the retina of each eye. Complications developed and he was not fully recovered when discharged.

Hundreds of otherwise healthy people have problems like these each year while skiing or climbing or hiking above 9,000 feet anywhere in the world. Scores die needlessly of such easily preventable illness. Thousands of people trek or climb in Nepal each year, and too many of them are sickened enough by altitude to turn back without completing their journey. Yet thousands of climbers have done technically difficult routes and stayed for weeks above 20,000 feet and even much higher without illness. Though far from as strong as at sea level, they have coped with lack of oxygen through the marvelously intricate adaptive processes which — given time — allow mountaineers to function remarkably well on the upper slopes of Everest breathing only the thin air about them.

Lack of oxygen also causes problems for a much larger population than climbers: hundreds of thousands of patients have chronic lung diseases like emphysema that prevent normal oxygenation of the blood and produce several signs and symptoms much like altitude illness. Not a few persons are knocked out and even permanently crippled or killed by accidents that impair their oxygen supply.

A woman unexpectedly developed respiratory arrest during a simple operation. Resuscitation was delayed and full respiration and circulation were not restored for about seven minutes. Though she survived, months later she was still unconscious.

An eighteen-year-old man injured in a car accident was brought to a hospital unconscious, barely breathing, and blue. Full oxygenation was restored after some difficulty, and he improved for a time, only to develop evidence of brain swelling and pulmonary edema and die twenty-four hours later.

A heavy smoker gradually developed shortness of breath and a cough over a period of many years and became partially disabled. Then he developed pneumonia involving more than half of his lungs. His condition deteriorated rapidly, and he became uncooperative and hostile, hallucinating badly, and sinking into a coma before he died.

A housewife, found unconscious from carbon-monoxide poisoning, showed evidence of brain damage and had hemorrhages in both eyes. She did not regain consciousness before dying from pulmonary and brain edema.

All these persons were affected by *hypoxia* (lack of oxygen). For some the problems came from going too fast to a potentially dangerous altitude. Others suffered because something interfered with their breathing or because they breathed air contaminated with a foreign gas. Healthy people have reached the highest point on earth breathing only the thin cold air about them — but only because they had taken weeks to acclimatize by slow ascent. Equally healthy people have died because they ascended too rapidly from sea level to 9,000 feet — an altitude barely noticeable to those who take time to adjust. At sea level people die rapidly if their oxygen supply is abruptly reduced by illness or injury, but thousands can tolerate the same low level of oxygen if their illness has come upon them gradually.

To fully appreciate why oxygen is essential to the life of mammals and how its lack affects almost every function, it is helpful to look at some fundamental physiology and to follow the stages by which oxygen reaches the living cells. Equally important are the mechanisms by which carbon dioxide — one product of metabolism — is cast out of the body and the subtle integrations by which the body acclimatizes. This review begins with a look at the evolution of our understanding of the physics of the atmosphere and the physiology of our bodies, for the story of man at altitude is interwoven with his exploration of the world about him and the world within.

Thousands of years ago, when the known world was limited to the horizon a man could see, survival depended on foraging and hunting, and it is not surprising that these early people had little time or reason to explore mountainous country where food and shelter were scarce and weather hostile. Just staying alive was a full-time job. Superstition or religion also kept people off the mountains. To the ancient Greeks mountains were home to many gods, and decent respect (and perhaps fear) kept them from intruding. Mount Olympus was the majestic home of Zeus, his wife Hera, and their multitude of children, and they feasted there on ambrosia between heroic (and often amorous) visits to the mortals below. Long before the Greeks, the patriarch Noah is reputed to have landed on top of 16,400-foot Mt. Ararat, the first and only mountaineer to have reached a summit by boat, under circumstances unlikely to recur. Legend describes him as miserably seasick, and perhaps with a hangover. But he was actually at sea level, so altitude — which does bother tourists who climb Ararat today — was not a problem.

Throughout the centuries many generations have lived on the high Tibetan plateau and in the Andes. Though we know of no permanent habitations above 17,000 feet anywhere in the world, a few caretakers have been living for several years at a mine at 20,000 feet in the Andes, and stone shrines and other relics found as high as 22,000 feet in the Andes strongly suggest that five centuries ago Andean man worked and worshipped there, if not permanently, at least for months at a time.

The Greek philosopher Empedocles was one of the early scientists curious enough to climb a high volcano — Mt. Etna, then probably higher than its present 10,000 feet. Legend has it that he leaped into the seething crater (some say to convince his followers of his divinity): the volcano he had come to study spewed out his brass slippers but kept the philosopher. One of his lasting contributions to science was his demonstration that air was compressible, which anticipated by 2,000 years further proof of such a revolutionary idea. Not many others in ancient Greece ventured high enough to notice the altitude, although Francis Bacon wrote:

The ancients had already noted that on the summit of Mount Olympus the air was so rare that in order to climb to it one must take with him sponges wet with vinegar and water and place them on the nostrils and mouth since the air, because of its rarity, did not suffice for respiration.

Bacon was quoting Livy, who referred to Aristotle, but there is no such statement about the rarity of high-altitude air in Aristotle's surviving works. Was this perhaps a very early observation that air is "thinner" at altitude, or did Livy or Bacon mean that it was more dry, or is it all a charming myth? Hippocrates, though he wrote a good deal about "good vapors" and "pestilential air" and their effect on health, does not mention altitude.

About the same time as Empedocles' leap, Xenophon was describing the Anabasis of Cyrus, during which he crossed many high mountain passes in Armenia, but he does not mention the effects of altitude, presumably being more occupied with hostile Armenians and Kurds and by hunger, thirst, and cold. Eighty years later, Alexander the Great made an even more perilous and longer journey, crossing higher passes, but no records survive to tell what he and his men may have endured from the altitude. In 218 B.C. Hannibal, the formidable Carthaginian general, crossed an alpine pass to overrun northern Italy, which believed itself secure behind the Alps. Just which pass his army with its 400 elephants did cross is uncertain, but all contenders for the honor are higher than 9,000 feet. Livy and Polybius, who described the campaign most vividly, wrote of cold and storm and avalanches that killed many elephants, but they did not mention the thin air at altitude.

Petrarch the great humanist seems to have made the first mountain ascent for pure pleasure, climbing Mont Ventoux (6,273 feet) in 1335, though other travelers preferred to look at mountains from as great a distance as possible and with fear. In 1178 Master John d'Bremble wrote of his crossing of the Great St. Bernard pass:

I have been on the Mount of Jove; on the one hand looking up to the heavens of the mountains, on the other shuddering at the hell of the valleys, feeling myself so much nearer heaven, I was sure my prayers would be heard. "Lord," I said, "restore me to my brethren that I may tell that they come not to this place of torment . . . where it is so slippery that you cannot stand . . . the death into which there is every facility for falling. . . ."

Peter, king of Aragon and Sicily and a true mountain climber, described his ascent of Pic Canigou (9,815 feet) in the Pyrenees: "On that mountain no man has ever lived nor has any son of man dared to ascend it, both on account of its excessive height and by reason of the difficulty and toil of the journey." The king had difficulties. His companions were terrified by the steepness and by thunder and lightning: "they threw themselves on the ground and lay there as it were lifeless" and implored the king to turn back. Then the two companions who remained "began to flag to such an extent that what with their weariness and their dread of the thunder they could scarcely breathe." Peter went on alone, and "when he was at the top of the mountain he found a lake there; and when he threw a stone into the lake a horrible dragon of enormous size came out of it and began to fly about in the air and to darken the air with its breath."

Explorers and trading caravans had been pushing over high

mountain passes in Central Asia for centuries, and some of their stories survive. One of the more complete describes the travels of Mirza Muhammad Haidar, who was born in Tashkent in A.D. 1500 and studied history as well as making it. He traveled extensively and gained firsthand knowledge of the high plateaus and great mountains of Central Asia. In a colorful chapter he describes some of the problems:

Another peculiarity of Tibet is the "dam-giri" which the Moghuls call "Yas."... The symptoms are a feeling of severe sickness, and in every case one's breath so seizes him that he becomes exhausted just as if he had run up a steep hill with a heavy burden on his back. On account of the oppression it causes, it is difficult to sleep. Should, however, sleep overtake one, the eyes are hardly closed before one is awoke with a start caused by oppression of the lungs and chest. ....When overcome by this malady the patient becomes senseless, begins to talk nonsense, and sometimes the power of speech is lost, while the palms of the hands and soles of the feet become swollen. Often when this last symptom occurs, the patient dies between dawn and breakfast time; at other times he lingers on for several days.... This malady only attacks strangers; the people of Tibet know nothing of it, nor do their doctors know why it attacks strangers.... The colder the air, the more severe is the form of the malady.... It is not peculiar to men, but attacks every animal that breathes, such as the horse.... One day, owing to the necessity of a foray, we had ridden faster than usual. On waking next morning I saw that there were very few horses in our camp and on inquiring I ascertained that more than 2000 had died during the night.... I have never heard of this disease outside of Tibet. No remedy is known for it.

Ney Elias, who translated this book in 1896, was one of the great Himalayan traveler-explorers of the last half of the nineteenth century, and added an interesting footnote:

In some respects he (Haidar) is at fault, as when he says that the natives do not suffer from "dam-giri." Tibetans born and bred at an elevation of, say, 12,500 feet, will suffer more severely from "dam-giri" (or dam as it is usually called) when they ascend to 17,000 or 18,000 feet, than natives of countries about the level of the sea. The degree of suffering depends on the constitution of the individual, or on how far he has become accustomed to high altitudes. . . . The malady is called . . . by the Indian population of the Himalaya "bish-ka-hawa" or "poisonous air." The Tibetan words are "dug-ri" or "poison of the mountain," and "la-dug" or "pass poison." . . . Mirza Haidar, when he prescribes the removal of the patient to the neighborhood of forts or villages, unconsciously proposes what is perhaps the only real cure — viz., a descent to a lower altitude.

The sixteenth century, though a time of great leaps of discovery in science and exploration, was also a period of religious conflict, war, superstition, and privation. Dragons and evil spirits were believed to live in the mountains, keeping all but the most venturesome from going high. One of the more detailed legends concerns Mt. Pilatus, named for Pontius Pilate, whose body was brought there after he had committed suicide in the Tiber and cast into a lake on the 9,000-foot summit. It was said that whenever the lake was disturbed, it overflowed and caused dreadful storms, floods, and even earthquakes. So real were such calamities that the local government in the fourteenth century strictly forbade anyone to even approach the lake; six clerics who did so in 1387 were severely punished. Conrad Gesner, scholar and physician, finally obtained permission to investigate the legend in 1585 and noted nothing abnormal, but not for another forty years did someone throw stones into the lake: nothing happened.

Gesner is the first European writer whose description of love for mountains and belief in their benefit to health has survived. In his book *On the Admiration of Mountains* he wrote:

I have determined . . . so long as the life divinely granted to me shall continue, each year to ascend a few mountains, or at least one, when the vegetation is flourishing, partly for the sake of suitable bodily exercise and the delight of the spirit. For how great the pleasure, how great think you are the joys of spirit touched as is fit it should be in wondering at the mighty mass of mountains while gazing upon their immensity and as it were in lifting one's head among the clouds. . . . I say therefore that he is an enemy of nature whosoever has not deemed lofty mountains to be worthy of great contemplation. . . . And so of all the elements in the variety of nature the supreme wonder resides in the mountains. In these it is possible to see "the burden of the mighty earth" just as if nature were vaunting herself and making trial of her strength by lifting to such height so great a weight.

Though a physician, he makes no mention of the unpleasant effects to be so vividly described by mountaineers still to come, and which, in fact during his lifetime, were being noted and would soon be described in another country and another tongue, by José d'Acosta. This intrepid Jesuit traveled throughout Peru, after the Conquistadores, and his account *The Natural and Moral History of the Indies,* written and published in 1590, some forty years after his travels, contains a graphic description of altitude illness:

There is in Peru, a high mountaine which they call Pariacaca, and having heard speake of the alteration it bred, I went as well prepared as I could according to the instructions which was given me by such as they call Vaguianos or expert men but not withstanding all my provision, when I came to mount the degrees, as they call them, which is the top of this mountaine I was suddenly surprised with so mortall and strange a pang, that I was ready to fall from the top to the ground: and though we were many in company yet everyone made haste (without tarrying for his companion), to free himself speedily from this ill passage. . . . I was surprised with such pangs of straining and casting as I thought to cast up my heart too; for having cast up meate fleugme, and choller, both yellow and greene; in the end I cast up blood with the straining of my stomacke. To conclude, if this had continued, I should undoubtedly have died. . . . Some in the passage demanded confession thinking verily to die . . . others left the ladders and went to the ground, being overcome with casting and going to the stoole: it was told to me that some have lost their lives there with this accident.

I beheld one that did beate himself against the earth, crying out for the rage and griefe which this passage of Pariacaca hadde caused. But commonly it doth no important harme, onely this, paine and troublesome distaste while it endures: and not onely the passage of Pariacaca hath this propertie, but also all this ridge of the mountaine which runnes above 500 leagues long, and in which place soever you passe

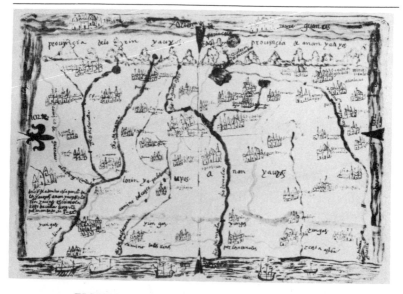

FIGURE 1. ACOSTA'S MAP OF PARIACACA

Father José d'Acosta has been called the Pliny of the New World because of his detailed description of all he saw during his missionary travels in the Andes. His vivid account of altitude illness is the earliest we have, but until recently it was not clear just where or how high the pass he calls Pariacaca actually was. Biochemist Dan Gilbert has painstakingly investigated this and I am indebted to him for use of this old map — not much perhaps for a journey, but the best available in general terms. Pariacaca, according to Gilbert, was the name given to a whole range of snowy mountains, and to one particular inn along a main road that crossed a 15,750-foot pass which can be identified today — and which was certainly high enough to make travelers sick. The pass is marked just below the dark circle at top center.

---

you shall find strange in temperatures, yet more in some parts than in other and rather to those which mount from the sea and from the plaines. . . .

For my part I holde this place to be one of the highest peaks of land in the worlde; for we mount a wonderful space. And in my opinion, the mountaine Nevade of Spaine, the Pirenees, and the Alpes of Italie, are as ordinarie houses, in regarde of hie Towers. I therefore perswade myselfe that the element of the air is there so subtile and delicate, as it is not proportionable with the breathing of man, which requires a more gross and temperate aire, and I beleeve it is the cause that doth so much alter the stomacke, & trouble all the disposition.

Dan Gilbert has examined maps of the Andes dating back to Acosta and concludes that Pariacaca was a well-traveled pass, almost 15,000 feet high, on the road from Lima to Jauja, near a mountain of the same name. From comparing several different translations of Acosta's book, he believes that Acosta also described the relative immunity to altitude shown by natives who came more slowly up the longer, more gradually rising eastern slopes, thereby taking time to acclimatize.

Acosta is the only participant in these adventures whose description of altitude sickness has survived, if any others were written. Cortés and Pizarro sent many of their men to craters on top of the Central American volcanoes to bring back sulfur to make gunpowder, but they left no record of their reaction to the altitude. They may have attributed any symptoms to the volcanic fumes, but more likely they were partially acclimatized from their long stay in the high valleys and their slow rate of climb.

In the Andes altitude sickness was familiar and called *puna* (literally meaning "high dry desert"), *mareo* ("sea sickness"), or *veta,* but whether all these names were of local origin or made up by the invaders is not clear. In Bolivia and Chile altitude sickness was called *soroche,* the Spanish word for antimony — and emanations from that ore were blamed for the symptoms. In other areas rhubarb plants, primroses, heather, or mosses were alleged to produce pestilential vapors that made men sick. There was general agreement that some places were worse than others — a belief that persists today!

The Incas may have recognized the effects of altitude sometime during the sixteenth century, for the Great Inca enforced laws controlling migration of his subjects between the sea coast and the high altiplano. Whether these were motivated by military, social, or political reasons or because of possible health effects is not clear.

As the fifteenth century ended and the glorious years of the Renaissance began, men were venturing farther across the oceans and higher onto the mountains and writing about the phenomena they observed. Acosta's long, detailed description of mountain sickness was followed in the next century by an explosion of scientific curiosity and exciting discoveries in physics, chemistry, anatomy, and physiology. At the same time, the great navigators crossed the oceans and more travelers penetrated high mountain ranges, crossed the deserts, and reported their sensations along with their discoveries. The Renaissance was a crowded, fertile, and exciting period of exploration — exploration of the physical universe and of the human body, and of their interrelationships.

Chapter Two

TOWARD UNDERSTANDING THE PHYSICAL UNIVERSE

ARISTOTLE'S LONG SHADOW fell over Europe for 1,500 years and effectively halted the growth of new ideas in science. His principles were fundamental to church doctrine, which held that the universe was static and perfect. But Aristotle's science was flawed by too much reliance on reason and too little experimental evidence. Looking toward the heavens, Aristotle could not conceive that space could be empty, because it would then have no dimensions. Light could not penetrate a space that did not exist, and therefore the stars could not be visible if a vacuum intervened between them and earth. At the same time he also argued that "in its own place every body has weight except fire, even air. It is proof of this that an inflated bladder weighs more than an empty one. . . ." Theologians, while agreeing with Aristotle that a vacuum did not exist, declared that it was certainly possible, because if God wished to create one he could surely do so.

Then like flowers at the end of a long winter, the arts and sciences burst into bloom as the Renaissance succeeded the Dark Ages. Suddenly, almost abruptly, established doctrines were challenged, and new ideas, freed from the shackles of the past, opened new vistas in physics, chemistry, medicine. It would almost seem that some ferment must have been loosed to catalyze so many fresh ideas in so many brilliant minds in so short a span of time.

Considering the difficulties of travel, it is remarkable how rapidly ideas spread across Europe, enabling a Dutchman, for example, to repeat and build upon the observations of a Paduan. Looking back on those inspiring times, it is clear that the great philosopher-scientists taught and learned from one another — and occasionally developed the same academic rivalries that scholars do today.

Not surprisingly, the nature of the universe, particularly the nature of the atmosphere, attracted great attention. Air and life and fire have been associated throughout recorded history, and the concept of "vital spirit" or "breath of life" goes back at least 4,000 years. The ancient Egyptians used a blowpipe to increase the heat of their furnaces; the Romans tested the safety of air at the bottom of a well by lowering into it a lighted candle, and Cicero appreciated the nourishment which the lungs drew from inspired air. Nevertheless, recognition that air has clearly definable physical properties was slow in coming, cramped by doctrinaire positions taken by many of the famous. One early dissenter was a Dutch philosopher, Isaac Beeckman, who wrote in his medical doctoral thesis in 1618: "It happens that air, in the manner of water, presses upon things and compresses them according to the depth of the super-incumbent air." He soon came into conflict with the famous French mathematician and religious philosopher René Descartes, who denied the possibility of a vacuum, while the great Italian scientist Galileo Galilei averred that air had no weight but was ambiguous about the existence of a vacuum! Beeckman was defiant: "for I admit nothing in philosophy, unless it is represented to the imagination as being perceptible to the senses." The controversy could not be settled by argument. As Beeckman said, experiments had to be done and data collected to prove one side or the other right.

During the first years of the seventeenth century some of the

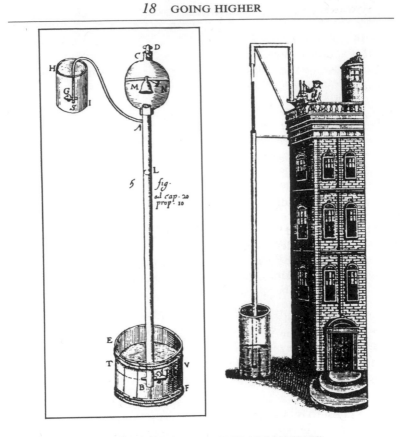

FIGURE 2. THE FIRST "BAROMETER"

Emmanuel Maignan, a close friend and associate of Gaspar Berti, left a detailed description of how Berti first demonstrated the effect of atmospheric pressure on a column of water:

> *This distinguished Gaspar . . . erected a rather long leaden tube (AB) on the wall of his house and made it secure. . . . The upper end (A) of the tube was opposite one of the windows . . . while the lower end (B) was not far from the ground and was provided with a brass tap or cock (R), this being within the cask (EF) filled with water for the purpose. To the upper end (A) was fitted . . . a glass vessel rather large but very solid, and having two necks and mouths, the wider one below into which the end of the tube was inserted at (A) as into a box; the narrower above at (C) made so it would fit the stem of the threaded brass screw (D). . . .*

This being made ready, the tap (R) closed and the cask (EF) filled with water . . . the entire tube as well as the glass vessel was filled from above through the opening (C). Then the opening (C) was closed with the screw (D) in order to seal the entire apparatus. . . .

At length when the tap (R) was opened the water flowed (contrary to the hope of many) out of the pipe into the cask (EF) to an easily observable height, but not all of it flowed out and it soon stood quite still . . . although the tap (R) had been open all the time. Then, when this tap (R) had been carefully closed again, the screw (D) was taken out above. And as soon as it was taken out behold! the air rushed in with a loud noise, filling the space previously abandoned by the water.

Later, using a sounding line, Berti determined that the water had stood in the tube eighteen cubits above the level of water in the cask, which Maignan remembered because it was the height that Galileo had observed was the most that water could rise in a suction pump or siphon.

At least ten years before this epochal demonstration, in 1630, Baliani, concluding like Beeckman that it was the existence of a vacuum which prevented water from being sucked or siphoned above a certain height, had written a long letter to Galileo pointing this out and at least seeming to suggest the experiment done by Berti.

Within a few years many others had repeated this experiment, and Torricelli was using honey, saltwater, wine, and finally mercury to develop what has become our modern barometer.

---

tools became available to make such studies. The microscope, the telescope, the clock, and the barometer and thermometer were all conceived and built in the space of a few decades. Of these, the barometer was the most crucial to studies of the atmosphere. Although it was no more possible for a Jesuit in 1640 to believe in the existence of a vacuum than for a scientist in 1940 to believe in the Indian rope trick, some had begun to challenge Aristotle with direct experiments. One of the early ones was a young Italian mathematician and astronomer named Gaspar Berti. He was very modest and left little record of what he did or why, so we rely on a more prolific philosopher, Emmanuel Maignan, who described the great experiment that Berti did in Rome about 1640, in the presence of a handful of friends, all scientists, all churchmen (see Figure 2).

A long leaden pipe was erected against the wall of Berti's house, with reservoirs and spigots at the lower and upper ends. When these were appropriately adjusted, water fell in the tube to a level some thirty feet above the level in the lower reservoir. Berti recognized that there must be a vacuum above this, in the top of the tube, which was exactly what he wished to show.

There was a good deal of quibbling over details before Evangelista Torricelli, a devoted student of Galileo's, heard of the experiment, immediately recognized its importance, and took the next important steps: he substituted mercury for water (which reduced the necessary tube from thirty feet to forty inches) and added a scale — which converted the device into a measuring instrument.

Priority in science is a will o' the wisp; few great ideas have sprung full-hatched from a single person, and each man climbs on the shoulders of his predecessors. The exact sequence of events in 1640–1645, who did what and when, and whose ideas inspired successive steps, is debated and not terribly important. Torricelli gave us the mercury barometer which, with many refinements, is the basic instrument we use today, and it is quite fitting that his name should be remembered in the units — torr — we now use, but at the same time, let us respect Gaspar Berti's imaginative experiment. In a famous letter of June 11, 1644, Torricelli wrote:

> *I have already hinted to you that some sort of philosophical experiment was being done concerning the vacuum; not simply to produce a vacuum, but to make an instrument which might show the changes in the air, now heavier and coarser, now lighter and more subtle.*

In one of these experiments, planned to determine the nature of the vacuum at the upper end of the tube, a mouse was placed in the lower reservoir and allowed to swim up through the mercury to the empty space. The mouse died, but it was not clear whether from struggling through the mercury or because of the vacuum.

These ideas were a giant leap forward: Torricelli thought

that with the instrument he hinted at he might be able to observe (and perhaps predict?) changes in weather, as Robert Boyle would do a few years later. But Torricelli went further and described the atmosphere, which he estimated might be fifty miles thick:

We live submerged at the bottom of an ocean of elementary air which is known by incontestable experiments to have weight, and so much weight, that the heaviest part near the surface of the earth weighs about one four hundredth as much as water.

There it is in a few short years: proof that a vacuum could exist, recognition of the weight of air, and a sensitive instrument with which to measure atmospheric pressure. Only three years after Bert's pioneering experiment, Otto Guericke (later made baron) invented an efficient vacuum pump and in a dramatic demonstration in Magdeburg showed conclusively how much pressure the atmosphere exerts on earth (see Figure 3). Word of these experiments spread rapidly through Europe.

In the fall of 1646 a physicist named Pierre Petit visited Blaise Pascal, one of the most distinguished French scientists, and together they repeated the Berti-Torricelli experiment. Pascal saw that there could be several explanations for the observed phenomena and determined to examine the questions further. Sometime later, in a letter (whose date has been the subject of heated controversy ever since), Pascal wrote to his brother-in-law Florin Perier:

I have imagined one decisive experiment that alone will fully enlighten us, if it can be executed with precision. It would mean repeating the experiments on vacuum several times in one day, in the same tube, with the same quicksilver, both at the foot and at the top of a mountain of at least 5–600 "toises,"* in order to establish whether the height of the quicksilver suspended in the tube is different or the same in the two situations. You no doubt already see that this experiment would decide the question, and that, if the height of the quicksilver is less at the top than at the bottom of the mountain (as I have reason to believe to be the case, even though all those that have thought about

---

* A "toise" is 6.9 feet.

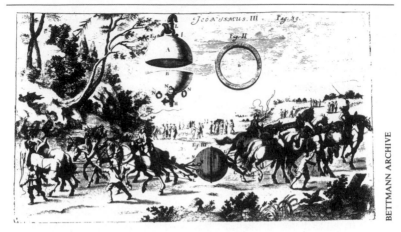

BETTMANN ARCHIVE

*FIGURE 3. GUERICKE DEMONSTRATES THE WEIGHT OF THE
ATMOSPHERE*

Controversy over the existence of a vacuum, suppressed for some time
by the traditions of the Church, was resolved early in the seventeenth century by several different approaches. One of these was Otto von Guericke's
use of the vacuum pump (which he had perfected) for an ingenious public
demonstration. Carefully fashioned hemispheres of heavy copper were
tightly fitted together and the air pumped out of the resulting sphere
known as the "Magdeburg sphere" for the town where this was first done.
Teams of horses attached to strong rings on each hemisphere could not
separate them, although they were not bolted but pressed together by atmospheric pressure. Later demonstrations used teams of strong men and
pulley systems for the same purpose during the years when Berti and others
confirmed the existence of a vacuum by demonstrating that the weight of
the "super-incumbent air" would raise liquid to a fixed height in a sealed
tube.

---

*this are contrary to this opinion), it will necessarily follow that the
weight and pressure of the air are the sole cause of this suspension of
the quicksilver, and not the horror of the vacuum, since it is quite obvious that there is much more weighing on the foot of the mountain than
on its summit; whereas one could not say that nature abhors a vacuum
at the foot of a mountain more than at the top.*

Then on September 18, 1648, came another great moment in the development of science when Florin Perier determined to test Pascal's idea and to measure the weight of air on the summit of a small mountain called Puy du Dôme (3,500 feet). At five that morning he assembled six highly trustworthy local dignitaries in the garden of the monastery in Clermont (see Figure 4). There "he took two similar glass tubes, hermetically sealed at one end, and repeated the Torricellian experiment." He filled both tubes with mercury, and then dexterously dipped each in the same vessel containing sixteen pounds of redistilled mercury, and observed that "the mercury level fell to the same height — twenty-six inches, three and one-half lines,* in each," leaving what we now know to be a near vacuum in the (sealed) upper end. To eliminate all doubt, he repeated the observation three times, and then, "leaving one tube set up at the monastery in charge of one of the monks who was to observe it frequently throughout the day," his distinguished party carried the other tube and the mercury up to the summit of Puy du Dôme, where he repeated the experiment:

The mercury stood at only twenty-three inches two lines. . . . Thus between the heights of quicksilver in these two experiments there was a difference of three inches and one and one-half lines; which ravished us all with admiration and astonishment and surprised us so much for our own satisfaction we wished to repeat it.

The party, though excited, was perhaps still skeptical and they made the experiment five times, each time getting identical results. Halfway down the mountain, using the same method, they found the level of mercury to be twenty-five inches. When they were assured back at the monastery that the height of mercury in that tube had been constant throughout the day, they knew they had for the first time demonstrated that the weight of air — the barometric pressure — decreases as alti-

* On most barometers of the day, an inch was divided into twelve parts or lines; three and one-half lines would thus be about one-third of an inch.

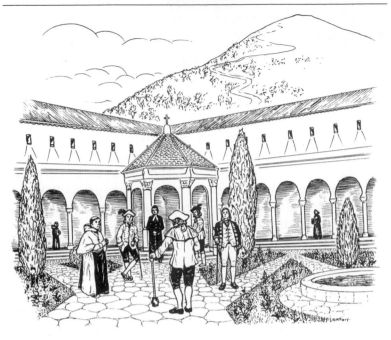

FIGURE 4. PERIER PREPARES TO CLIMB THE PUY DU DÔME

Florin Perier measured the barometric pressure at the bottom and on the summit of the Puy du Dôme, and showed that it decreased as altitude increased.

tude increases. This experiment, so simple to our modern eyes, was a great triumph for Pascal, by then sickly and turning from science to religion.

By 1660 Robert Boyle had repeated Berti's experiment (also using a long water-filled tube attached to his house, if the illustration in his book is accurate) and made many types of mercury barometers. He showed that barometric pressure decreased with increasing height, and seems to have been the first to use changes in barometric pressure to predict changes in weather. An extraordinary series of experiments confirmed an observation made by Beeckman that the volume of a gas decreased as the pressure on it was increased — a law that bears Boyle's name today although his assistant and later colleague Robert Hooke did most of the experiments and first elucidated the "law."

Many others were conducting similar studies throughout Europe, and it became clear very rapidly that air had weight and was compressible and thus the atmospheric weight or pressure was lower the higher one went. Boyle read Acosta's writings and his curiosity was piqued. He made inquiries of a number of travelers who had crossed high passes and of others who lived among mountains: all agreed that breathing was more difficult at altitude, and Boyle concluded that this was due to thin air, as Acosta had speculated.

These great scientist-philosophers of the seventeenth century still believed the Aristotelian doctrine that the universe was made of four elements — fire, water, earth, and air — even though Paracelsus had somewhat earlier begun questioning this concept as he generated a new kind of "air" (hydrogen) from iron filings and acid and showed that it burned violently. Paracelsus conceived of a kind of spirit which he called "the archaeus" that drew particles of matter together. By then a number of basic elements like sulfur, mercury, and iron were already known, though not yet seen as building blocks for other substances. The Belgian Johann Baptista van Helmont (who died after thirteen years of torture by the Inquisition because of his beliefs) used a new word, *gas,* to describe a state of matter separate from solids and liquids, probably drawing from the German *Geist,* or "spirit." Helmont described several new gases and proposed a theory of combustion that later led to the phlogiston theory, which influenced studies of the atmosphere for more than a century.

After serving Boyle for several years, Robert Hooke was appointed curator of the newly formed Royal Society and soon was charged with bringing to the meetings a number of new experiments each week. Boyle was one of the more active contributors, and during an incredibly productive five-year period,

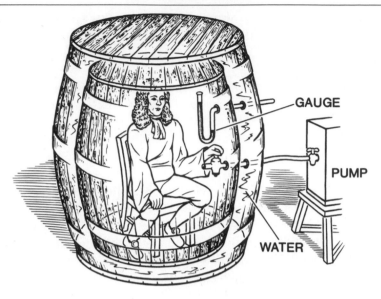

GAUGE

PUMP

WATER

FIGURE 5. ROBERT HOOKE'S "DECOMPRESSION CHAMBER"

As soon as Robert Boyle heard of Guericke's vacuum pump, he and his then-assistant Robert Hooke made their own "New Pneumatical Engine" and examined the effects of a partial vacuum on all sorts of animals, minerals, and vegetables. In December 1670, after many reports to the Royal Society, Hooke proposed "a new way of making a vessel for extracting air, so large, that a man might fit in it, and so contrived, as to rarefy the air to a certain degree...." He was instructed to proceed, and on February 2, 1671,

> ... *being asked, whether the air-vessel for a man to fit in was yet ready, answered that it was.... Being asked, how it was contrived, he said, that it consisted of two tuns, one included in the other; the one to hold a man, the other filled with water to cover the former, thereby to keep it staunch; with tops to put on with cement; or to take off; one of them having a gage, to see to what degree the air is rarefied; as also a cock to be turned by the person who sits in the vessel....*

A month later he reported

> ... *that he himself had been in it, and by the contrivance of bellows and valves blown out of it one-tenth part of the air (which he found by a gage suspended within the vessel) and had felt no inconvenience but that of some pain in his ears at the breaking out of the air included in them, and the like pain upon the readmission of the air pressing the air inward.*

Hooke's courageous experiment is undoubtedly the first time a man was "taken up" in a decompression chamber, and this along with all his other studies of air and pressure should give him a prominent place in altitude physiology. The illustration is as close as my illustrator and I could come from the above description included in a *History of the Royal Society,* reprinted in 1967 in Brussels. Curiously, I could find no mention of this experiment in Hooke's book *Curious Philosophical Observations and Experiments,* where he describes many experiments with increased and decreased atmospheric pressure, or in Boyle's works.

Hooke and Boyle produced some of the most ingenious and important studies of the composition of air that had yet been made. One of the more famous caused a great deal of confusion: when a mouse and a lighted candle were placed under a bell jar, the candle went out long before the mouse died, which led to the concept that life and combustion might be different. Though Hooke opposed this view, he received little support. The Society observed all sorts of experiments: mice, snakes, shellfish, birds, flowers, plants, and insects were all studied under the bell jar, or in flasks evacuated by the "New Pneumatical Engine" built by Hooke but based on the vacuum pump first made by Guericke around 1647.

After these experiments on animals began to pall, Hooke was directed by the Royal Society to make a vessel big enough to hold a man while it was evacuated! There was some delay, and at several meetings members expressed impatience, but finally the device was ready, and Hooke entertained the members in his rooms. He entered the inner barrel, and the "New Pneumatical Engine" extracted about one-tenth of the air, taking him to a simulated altitude of about 3,000 feet (see Figure 5). He noticed no discomfort other than slight pressure in his ears, but this first decompression-chamber experiment on man was not repeated, and the Society went on to other subjects.

Boyle was developing his own ideas of the composition of air:

. . . the atmospherical air consists of three different kinds of corpuscles . . . first, these numberless particles . . . in the form of vapors . . . the second more subtle consists of those exceedingly minute atoms the magnetical effluvia of the earth . . . the third sort is its characteristic and essential property, I mean permanently elastic parts.

He outlined a program of studies which might well have led to a true understanding of combustion had he been able to complete them, but he turned to other interests. Another brilliant contemporary took up the work. John Mayow, who had become first a lawyer, then a physician, was attracted by a new theory, probably first proposed by the Dane Olaus Borrichius (also called Ole Borch), that air contained a special life-giving substance much as Helmont had postulated. In 1678 Borch actually generated this substance, which we now know to be oxygen, by the decomposition of potassium nitrate, but failed to appreciate the significance of his discovery.

Advances in instrumentation had been keeping pace with theories and expanded opportunities for experimental proofs. One of these was the improvement in glass making — a process known for several thousand years but only in this period brought to a specialized skill kept secret by the Venetians at Murano. Reliable laboratory glassware permitted more accurate volumetric measurements, and the concurrent evolution of very sensitive analytical balances made possible precise measurement of weight lost or gained by combustion, for example. Technology was ready for the next great leap ahead.

John Mayow used these advances to make his major contributions. He soon appreciated that the atmosphere consisted of at least two kinds of gases: "nitro-aerial particles are necessary for the support of life and . . . combustion; while the other, remaining after this constituent has been removed, is incapable of supporting either life or combustion." His theories were backed by careful experiments. In 1674 he wrote: "I take it for granted that the air contains certain particles termed by us elsewhere nitro-aerial which are absolutely indispensable for the production of fire."

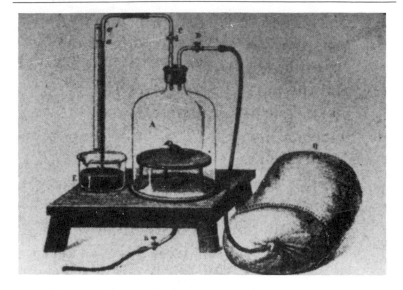

FIGURE 6. LIFE IN A VACUUM: THE BENEFITS OF OXYGEN

John Mayow tried to determine the composition of air by watching the extinction of a candle (or the death of a small bird or mouse) within a sealed bell jar, concluding in 1674 that some element in air was essential for "combustion." Later a vacuum pump was used to prove that low pressures too were incompatible with life in experiments such as that shown above. Pressure was measured by the changes in mercury level in the U-shaped glass gauge. Soon larger containers were used, eventually evolving into the steel "bell" used by Bert. The modern counterpart is a huge "room" sometimes accommodating 15–25 persons, and capable of reaching 50,000 feet or more in simulated low pressure. Just a hundred years after Mayow, Lavoisier repeated his work, adding oxygen to the bell jar and showing that a mouse or bird lived longer in the enriched gas, confirming Mayow's belief that some "vital spirit" in air was necessary for life. Lavoisier named the new gas "oxygine," and Priestley, who had publicly reported similar work shortly before Lavoisier, breathed some of the gas himself, writing that he fancied he perceived a peculiar lightness to his breathing. These studies laid the foundation for Paul Bert's important studies. He was able to make bags of leather to contain oxygen and showed that this sustained life in animals kept under evacuated bell jars (*above right*), and also prevented or relieved his own symptoms in the decompression chamber.

He showed this by burning a candle under a bell jar sealed with water and watching the water level rise as the candle burned out, just as Helmont had done many years earlier. He carried this experiment one exciting step forward:

Let a small bell jar in which a little animal say a mouse has been put be accurately applied to a tightly stretched skin to form a seal. When things have been arranged in this manner, it will in a short time be seen that the jar is firmly fixed to the skin, and the skin also at the place where it lies under the jar is forced upwards into the cavity of the glass just as if the jar had been applied with a flame enclosed in it. And this will take place while the animal is still breathing. From this it is clear that the elastic power of the air enclosed in the aforesaid jar has been diminished by the breathing of the animal so that it is no longer able to resist the pressure of the surrounding air.

After many experiments, Mayow was satisfied:

And in fact I have ascertained from experiments with various animals that the air (in the sealed jar) is reduced in volume by about one-fourteenth by the breathing of the animal.

And further:

From what has been said it is quite certain that animals in breathing draw from the air certain vital spirits. . . . That nitro-aerial spirit is by means of respiration transmitted into the mass of the blood and the fermentation and heating of the blood are produced by it.

Not for another hundred years would so clear a statement of the essential role of oxygen in supporting life be formulated. Some feel that Mayow deserves credit for identifying the importance of oxygen to life and combustion — a concept that would not come for another century, but to history he remains one of the background contributors.

Today we are so accustomed to the headlong pace of science, and the apparently endless flow of new ideas and inventions tumbling over one another faster than we can absorb or use them, that the developments of the first century of the Renaissance might seem slow and obvious. But consider what took place from 1550 to 1650: the Aristotelian theory was refuted and the existence of a vacuum proven. That the atmosphere which envelops earth had weight and was compressible was not only proven, but changes in atmospheric pressure with altitude were measured. And the *"spiritus mundi,"* or aether, on which life depends had been recognized to be a mixture of gases, one of which was essential to life and combustion. Many of the scientist-philosophers turned experimenters and began to prove in the laboratory what their predecessors had merely hypothesized. Torricelli and Berti, Pascal and Perier, Borch and Helmont, and Boyle and Mayow had built a set of giant steps toward understanding the world they lived in. For each of these there were many others whose names are today almost unknown (Baliani, for example) who also contributed, sometimes long before those who are now so famous.

Near the end of the seventeenth century a chemist, J. J. Becher, encouraged one of his students, Georg Ernst Stahl, to study Borch's concept of a special life-supporting substance in air. Stahl soon postulated that all substances which could be burned were compounds, one part of which was an odorless invisible gas which he christened "phlogiston," or "fire-substance." He theorized that when something burned, this principle was released and the substance became "dephlogisticated." But the delicate scales by then available showed that some substances gained rather than lost weight by combustion. Stahl tried to explain this by theorizing that phlogiston had a property the opposite of weight, that is, the quality of levity, so that as this negative weight escaped, the compound became heavier. Though there were demonstrable flaws in this theory, it prevailed for over a century and engaged the minds of some of the most brilliant scientists of the time.

One of these, Joseph Black, became Professor of Chemistry at Edinburgh in the mid–eighteenth century and was thought the most eloquent teacher of his time. Students copied his lectures word for word and he read his classes the identical lectures for twenty-five years. In one he demonstrated a new gas, "fixed air," which we know as carbon dioxide. He described this as "a sort of air quite distinct from common air, though it is commonly mixed with it in small quantity." He showed that this different gas was heavier than air and could be poured from one container to another, that it was formed by burning, that it was present in the exhaled air, and that it was a major constituent of "choke damp," the bane of miners. His was the first series of clear and well-planned experiments where everything was carefully measured and nothing was taken on trust. Daniel Rutherford and later Henry Cavendish continued his studies, and Cavendish supported the phlogiston theory for several years after all others had abandoned it, arguing that hydrogen, which he showed to be lighter than air in 1766, was phlogiston. Much effort in the first half of the eighteenth century went to the studies of his curious concept, but it was scarcely wasted.

Oxygen is so central to life and to any discussion of altitude illness that the tangled and controversial story of its birth (or perhaps its delivery) deserves a little more than passing mention, even though the "facts" seem to depend somewhat on the nationality or the biases of the reporter. The gas was actually made in the late seventeenth century by Ole Borch, but he did not realize what he had done and did not pursue the finding. Then between 1770 and 1773 a Swedish pharmacist, Carl Wilhelm Scheele, after an extraordinary and systematic series of experiments, not only generated oxygen from saltpeter, but even though young had the courage to point out shortcomings in the popular phlogiston theory of combustion, which of course did not endear him to his elders. He called his new gas "vitriol air" but soon changed this to "fire air" when he realized it was essential for combustion. Though primarily a chemist, he was also much interested in physiology and botany, and made many significant experiments in these fields as well.

In France, during this same time, Antoine-Laurent Lavoisier was doing similar experiments. Unlike his British rival Priestley, Lavoisier came from a well-to-do family and after an excellent education devoted himself to science from an early age. By 1772, though only twenty-eight years old, he made experiments he considered important enough to prompt this letter to the French Academy:

> *As this discovery appears to me to be one of the most interesting which has been made since the time of Stahl, I thought it expedient to secure myself the property by depositing the present note in the hands of the Secretary of the Academy, to remain secret until the period when I shall publish my experiments.*

On September 30, 1774, Scheele wrote Lavoisier to thank him for a book and in the letter (only recently uncovered) described how oxygen might be made. Lavoisier was interested and, as his laboratory notes show, used Scheele's instructions to supplement experiments he had been conducting for several years. It seems likely he was also spurred by the fact that a summary of Scheele's experiments had been published early in 1772, though Scheele's book, delayed by the procrastination of a colleague, did not appear until August 1777, three years after the generally accepted "birthday" of oxygen. Lavoisier also knew that another inquisitive and imaginative scientist was also on the trail.

Joseph Priestley was a theologian whose interest in chemistry was apparently stimulated by Hermann Boerhaave's textbook in 1755 and led to his teaching the subject a few years later. This interest in chemistry, particularly in gases, lasted the rest of his life, and his efforts climaxed in the fall of 1774.

On Saturday, November 19, he set up his crucial experiment, but on Sunday, preoccupied with his duties as a minister, he did not work in his laboratory. On Monday, November 21, 1774, he placed some mercuris calcinatus (red lead or mercuric oxide) in a closed glass vessel and heated it, obtaining about an ounce of vapor, which he carefully transferred to another container. Then:

In this air as I had expected, a candle burned with a valid flame. . . .
In ignorance of the real nature of this kind of air I continued from this
time to the first of March following. I procured a mouse and put it into
a glass vessel containing two ounce measures of the air obtained from
mercuris calcinatus. Had it been common air, a full grown mouse such
as this was would have lived in it about a quarter of an hour. In this air
however my mouse lived a full half hour.

Priestley was well aware of the limitations of animal experiments, apparently, and he proceeded cautiously:

I did not certainly conclude that this air was any better, because
though one mouse would live only a quarter of an hour in a given
quantity of air, I knew it was not impossible but that another mouse
might have lived in it half an hour. [So he] procured another mouse,
and putting it into less than two ounce measures of air extracted from
mercuris calcinatus . . . I found it lived three-quarters of an hour.
Being now fully satisfied of the superior goodness of this kind of air I
proceeded to measure that degree of purity with as much accuracy as I
could.

This he did quite ingeniously by mixing what he called
"dephlogisticated air" with "nitrous air," which was nothing
more than room air in his laboratory. He titrated the capacity of his new air to support life and combustion by testing
different mixtures, and then, bravely and prophetically, he
continued:

My reader will not wonder, that, after having ascertained the supe-
rior goodness of dephlogisticated air by mice living in it, and the other
tests above mentioned, I should have the curiosity to taste it myself. I
have gratified that curiosity, by breathing it, drawing it through a
glass-syphon, and, by this means, I reduced a large jar full of it to the
standard of common air. The feeling of it to my lungs was not sensibly
different from that of common air; but I fancied that my breast felt
peculiarly light and easy for some time afterwards. Who can tell
but that, in time, this pure air may become a fashionable article in
luxury. Hitherto only two mice and myself have had the privilege of
breathing it.

Scheele in Sweden was writing at about the same time:

. . . our atmosphere ought not to be considered as a simple fluid substance, for, when freed from all heterogeneous admixture, it is found . . . to consist of two very different kinds of air; the one is called corrupted air, *because it is very dangerous and fatal, as well as to living animals as vegetables; it constitutes the greatest part of our atmosphere. The other is called* pure air, fire air. *This kind of air is* salutary, supports respiration, *and consequently the circulation; without it we could form no distinct idea, either of fire, or how it is kindled. It constitutes but the smallest part of the whole atmosphere. Now as we know this air is of the most immediate necessity for the support of our health.*

The experiments which he carried out during 1778 and 1779 led him to conclude:

Our atmosphere, therefore, contains always, though with some little difference, nearly the same quantity of pure or fire air, 27%, which is a very remarkable fact; and to assign the cause of it seems difficult, as a quantity of pure air, in supporting fire, daily enters into a new union; and a considerable quantity of it is likewise corrupted, or changed into aerial acid, as well by plants as by respiration; another fresh proof of the great care of our Creator for all that lives.

Although Lavoisier had been working toward oxygen for a long time, one cannot help suspecting that he was hurried by the letter from Scheele and by a meeting with Priestley — both of which showed that others were nearing the same prize he sought.

At any rate, Lavoisier described his experiments in a paper read to the French Academy on April 26, 1775, five weeks after Priestley's report, and in 1789 published in his great textbook of chemistry, among many other studies, details of the experiment that had led him to oxygen:

I introduced four ounces of pure mercury into the [container] and, by means of a siphon exhausted the air so as to raise the quicksilver level, and I carefully marked the height at which it stood by pasting on

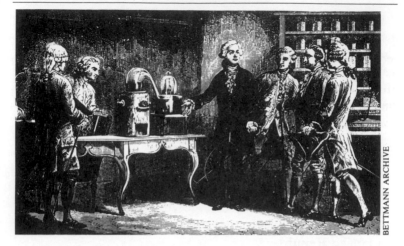

BETTMANN ARCHIVE

FIGURE 7. LAVOISIER IN HIS LABORATORY

Antoine-Laurent Lavoisier was a brilliant chemist, and although he did not originate the experiments which led to the isolation of oxygen, he shares with Priestley credit for most of the final work. Here he is demonstrating the distillation of mercury to his colleagues. In order to obtain the hydrogen which he needed for the newly developed Charlière balloons, he decomposed water into hydrogen and oxygen by percolating water through rings in a large gun barrel heated to incandescence! Ingenious though this method was, it proved impracticable for the generation of the large volumes needed, and balloonists soon turned to chemical sources. Lavoisier's laboratory was a gathering place for many distinguished scientists, and his textbook of chemistry remained a classic for many years.

---

a slip of paper. . . . I lighted a fire in the furnace which I kept almost continually burning twelve days so as to keep the quicksilver always very near the boiling point. Nothing remarkable took place during the first day; the mercury, though not boiling, was continually evaporating. . . . At the end of twelve days . . . I extinguished the fire and allowed the vessel to cool . . . the remaining air . . . had lost about one-sixth of its bulk and was no longer fit either for respiration or for combustion. Animals being introduced into it were suffocated in a few seconds and when a taper was plunged into it, it was extinguished as if it had been immersed in water.

Both Priestley and Lavoisier were giants in their time and their places in history are assured on many counts. They were also competitors in a great race and to some degree antagonists. Priestley clung to the phlogiston theory to the end of his life, although he insisted he would abandon it were he convinced that it was wrong. Lavoisier too was reluctant to abandon phlogiston until his demonstration that water was made up of hydrogen and oxygen; he was then convinced that his "oxygine" was a separate element, essential to life and combustion.

Both were versatile scientists and social reformers. Priestley supported the French Revolution, while Lavoisier was put to death in 1794 by a revolutionary tribunal. Though the comment "The Republic has no need for chemists" attributed to the judge who condemned him is apocryphal, a witness to the execution said more tellingly: "It took only an instant to cut off that head and a hundred years may not produce another like it."

By the end of the century it was clear that a portion of the ambient air supported life and combustion while the remainder was inert. The phlogiston theory was effectively eliminated by Lavoisier's demonstrations and by Priestley — though Priestley never fully renounced it. Several questions arose: Was this vital air, this "oxygine," present in all air everywhere? Was it constant in amount or did it differ from place to place? And most important — bearing in mind the candle and mouse experiment that had puzzled the Royal Society a century before — if "burning" and "living" were similarly dependent on oxygen, why did not the generated heat burn up the living tissues? It would be almost another century before this question was answered.

The experiments of Scheele, Lavoisier, and Priestley were repeated in many parts of Europe and on the summits of low mountains with the same results — about one-fifth of the air was oxygen. John Dalton, an imaginative scientist who revived the ancient atomic theory of Democritus, after ingenious studies and hypotheses advanced the law which now bears his name: "The total pressure exerted by a mixture of gases is equal to the sum of the pressures of the different gases making up the mixture, each gas acting separately and independently of the others." This "law of partial pressures" governs all of our theories and observations relating to respiration and was a major contribution to scientific progress. How simple this sounds today and how obvious, yet what immense imagination and painstaking experimentation was necessary to reach these conclusions. Advances came with a rush and in clusters, rather than as a steady flow. The names of the giants survive, but one wonders how many others had flashes of inspiration and made new discoveries only to be, through some quirk of time or publicity, "unwept, unhonored, and unsung."

Meanwhile the oceans and continents were being explored as well. Conrad Gesner and Professor Marti made their annual pilgrimages onto the mountains for pleasure. Domp Julian de Beaupré, in the same year that Columbus sailed to the New World, was ordered by the king of Spain (apparently on a whim) to climb a formidable rock pinnacle — Mont Aiguille (7,000 feet) — the first major rock climb. That there were many other mountain travelers and explorers then is suggested by the popularity of a remarkable book by Josias Simler published in 1574. Titled *De Alpibus Commentarius,* it could be described as the first Baedeker guide, cataloguing just about all one would want to know about mountain journeys. Simler described the dangers of avalanches and rockfalls, storms and the hazards of traveling on snow-covered glaciers. He included remarkable descriptions of the various aids to climbing used in his time and much like those of today — crampons, ice axes, and ladders. He advised the use of ropes on glaciers and described what we now call hypothermia, an insidious sleep brought on by cold and often leading to death. Commercial travelers must have found invaluable his advice about the food and lodging to be found in remote villages. Simler makes no mention of mountain sickness . . . nor of dragons.

Conrad Gesner, one of the earliest to proclaim his love of mountains, published seventy-two books in his lifetime and had no less than eighteen in manuscript when he died at the age of forty-nine during an epidemic of plague in 1565. One of his most ambitious efforts was an inventory of all the known animals — including descriptions of 250 varieties of dragons. An even more comprehensive work was undertaken by Ulisse Aldrovandi, an Italian naturalist and physician, but only four volumes were published between 1559 and his death in 1605; nine more appeared in the next fifty years. Aldrovandi too took dragons seriously, and indeed they were taken for granted even as late as 1712 when a distinguished Swiss professor, Johann Jakob Scheuchzer, made a systematic catalogue of them, apparently led to the study through his passion for paleontology, a field which he is said to have originated.

Scheuchzer was born in 1672, wrote an immense number of scientific works, and traveled extensively throughout the Alps. For several years he took sworn depositions from "persons of good character and repute" who had seen or, in some cases, even been attacked by dragons in mountainous areas. He described and painted these beasts very carefully: they came in several sizes, some had wings but no feet while others had feet but no wings, and some had long tails. Some breathed fire and smoke, and some were very small — not much larger than a dog. Were these eyewitness accounts like those many thousands of "reliable" sightings of unidentified flying objects that have made *UFO* part of our language? What did these persons of good repute and character actually see?

Did the fear of dragons keep men from the mountains? Perhaps attractions like rock crystals, topaz, and amethyst or game like chamois overcame anxiety over dragons, because some did climb and explore, and of course certain passes like the Great St. Bernard had been used for many generations. Nevertheless, fear of the unknown — including dragons—was more common than altitude illness.

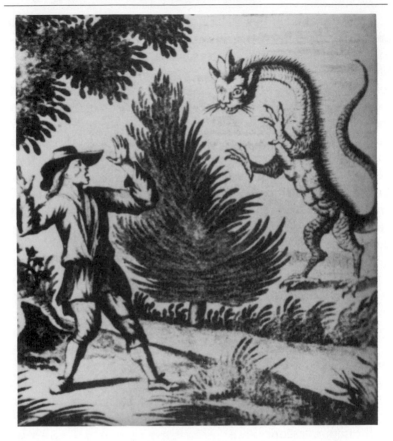

*FIGURE 8. THERE WERE (ALLEGEDLY) DRAGONS
ON THE MOUNTAINS*

Scheuchzer patiently collected many affidavits from persons who had actually seen — or even claimed to have been attacked by — dragons in the Alps and made many drawings of them. Probably fear of dragons as well as other superstitions did keep many people from climbing in the sixteenth and seventeenth centuries, but there was also cold and storm to deter them. Are these stories and pictures any more unbelievable than our contemporaries' reports of the Loch Ness monster, or UFOs, or visitors from outer space?

A sleepy little hamlet in the French Alps was the scene of the first major mountaineering efforts. In 1741 Windham and Pococke, with nine British companions, visited the valley below Mont Blanc and published a small booklet describing its splendors. Tourists were soon attracted by that magnificent snow-covered mountain, the highest in Europe, among them an artist named Marc-Theodore Bourrit, who made many paintings of the valley and the lovely mountain. He later made four attempts to climb it, once coming within a few hundred feet of the 15,400-foot summit before turning back because of illness (from altitude?). Bourrit was an artist and amateur climber, not a scientist like the man whose name is most often and widely associated with Mont Blanc: Horace-Bénédict de Saussure.

De Saussure first visited Chamonix in 1760 at the age of twenty, just two years before being appointed Professor of Philosophy at Geneva National Academy. He was the first of the great scientist-mountaineers drawn to high peaks by both these loves. In 1760 he offered a substantial reward to the first person to reach the summit, and two years later the first serious attempt was made by a local named Pierre Simon. Eight more attempts were made before a Chamonix doctor, François Paccard, and a local guide, Jacques Balmat, reached the summit on August 8, 1786. They were carefully watched from the valley through telescopes, but it was impossible to tell which of the two first stepped on the actual top, which led to an ugly controversy for many years. They made no mention of altitude illness. During the next forty years, according to Auldjo, who in 1828 published one of the most beautiful histories of Mont Blanc, there were fourteen successful ascents, fewer than take place in one week today, and a larger but unrecorded number of failures. De Saussure made the third ascent in 1787, after his two previous attempts, one with Bourrit, had failed. He spent four hours on top, later writing a vivid description of his misery from the altitude: "I myself who am so accustomed to the

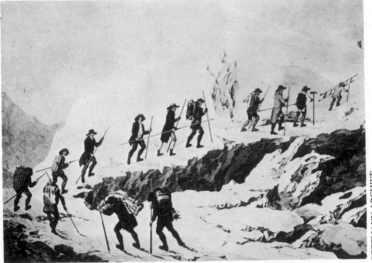

BETTMANN ARCHIVE

FIGURE 9. DE SAUSSURE ON MONT BLANC:
THE FIRST SCIENTIST-CLIMBER

De Saussure loved Mont Blanc for its beauty and for the challenge it offered to the daring; his first attempts on the summit failed, but on August 3,
1787, with a large party of guides led by Balmat (who had made the first
ascent in 1786 and the second earlier in 1787), he reached the summit. His
guides (pictured here in a contemporary painting) were burdened with scientific equipment even on this pioneering venture, for de Saussure was primarily a man of science, and he made many observations of the weather,
temperature, snow conditions, and especially of the physiological reactions
of himself and his companions (including his valet, who had never before
been on a mountain). He continued these studies for several years on other
peaks in the range of Mont Blanc, and his records are the first major scientific contribution to the study of high altitude.

air of the mountains, who feel better in this air than in that of
the plain, was completely exhausted." And when he tried to
conduct his various experiments:

I was constantly forced to interrupt my work and devote myself en-
tirely to breathing. . . . The kind of fatigue which results from the rar-

ity of the air is absolutely unconquerable; when it is at its height, the most terrible danger would not make you take a single step further.

De Saussure made observations of pulse and respiration on many summits and compared these readings with those made in the valleys. His travels and experiments were published between 1786 and 1796 in four volumes titled *Voyages dans les Alpes.* On one trip he journeyed up the great glacier above Chamonix, known as the Mer de Glace, to the Col du Géant, an 11,000-foot pass leading to Italy, and stayed there for several days. This was particularly daring because contemporaries believed that even a single night at so great a height would be fatal. Instead he enjoyed himself greatly, and carried on his experiments for two days, being forced to leave only when it was found that his guides had ransacked the supplies and left him without wine.

For several decades climbers attempted Mont Blanc with some success, and the mountain became world famous in 1852 due to a young physician, Albert Smith, who reached the top in 1851, and gave a well-advertised public lecture in March of the following year profusely "illustrated by a brilliant series of Dioramic Views painted expressly from the original sketches." Smith was such an instant success he left medicine for show business, giving nightly accounts of his ascent for six years. His detailed description was reasonably accurate on facts, and the paintings were dramatic. Although trained as a physician, Smith did not contribute to the science of altitude except indirectly. His companions on the climb described him as

. . . utterly exhausted. He passed two nights (during the climb) almost without sleep and this, with lack of appetite, dispirited him. He was walking fast asleep with his eyes open, with strange illusions that people he knew in London were following and calling after him.

Was he perhaps suffering from brain edema, a form of altitude illness? A cup of champagne on the summit revived him.

Smith undoubtedly stimulated hundreds of tourists to visit

the Alps, particularly Mont Blanc, but a few true mountaineers were already making spectacular climbs throughout the Alps. They founded the Alpine Club, still today the doyen of mountaineering excellence, whose annual journal carries the subtitle "A Record of Mountain Adventure and Scientific Observation." Though few of the early articles mention mountain sickness, a member named Joanne wrote in the *Journal* in 1872:

> *The lightness and great rarity of air in the Alps . . . cause at certain altitudes very noticeable physiological phenomena such as . . . nausea, drowsiness, panting, headache, fatigue, etc.; some of these symptoms even compel certain individuals to turn back as soon as they have reached 3,000 meters.*

Paul Bert, generally regarded as the father of high-altitude physiology, commented in 1877:

> *If these symptoms are so frequent . . . why not mention them in accounts which are often so prolix and loaded with uninteresting details. We must confess their importance and severity have been so exaggerated that travellers affected only by panting and palpitations are willing to deny even the reality of an illness they read so much in advance . . . most of the tourists whose narratives fill the Alpine Journal have hardly any scientific interest in their ascents; they climb for the sake of climbing . . . they are almost afraid of being ridiculed for mountain sickness as they are for seasickness.*

On the other hand, there was a time when failure to record the agonies of mountain sickness cast some doubt on the validity of the summit claim.

During this golden age of alpine climbing (1850–1875) virtually all of the alpine peaks were climbed, and on many the usual route led to the opening up of more difficult alternatives. Most climbers were from the leisured or professional class in England: geologists, physicians, or university faculty. Though they climbed for adventure and excitement, the scientifically minded described their symptoms at altitude, while others evolved theories to define the motion of glaciers and formation of mountains. Before long, mountain climbers were traveling all over the world in search of new peaks to conquer, and their observations contributed greatly to what scientists like Angelo Mosso and Paul Bert would soon learn about high-altitude physiology.

Chapter Three

EXPLORATION OF THE HEAVENS

Just how high above earth did the atmosphere extend? Did it end abruptly or gradually? What lay beyond? Even before Berti and Torricelli, others whose names are less known today had come close to the truth. One of them was Giovanni Baliani, who wrote two important letters to Galileo Galilei in 1630. In the first he respectfully offered an explanation (which happens to be correct) of why siphons function only if they are less than a certain height. Galileo answered rather condescendingly that the explanation lay in a force unique to the vacuum (about which the great man was ambiguous). In his second letter Baliani suggested (quite deferentially) that air had weight and that the higher one went, the lighter it would be, the same conclusion Beeckman had reached a dozen years earlier almost unnoticed.

Fourteen years later Torricelli was more specific:

Then writers have observed regarding the twilight that the vaporous air is visible above us for about fifty or fifty-four miles. But I do not think it is as much as this because I should then admit that the vacuum ought to produce a much greater resistance than it does.

First Perier and later the experiments that Robert Boyle arranged at different places throughout Europe confirmed Baliani's prediction and Torricelli's beliefs: air did get thinner and pressed less heavily on the earth the higher one went. A century and a half would elapse before the identification of oxygen and the demonstration that wherever it was measured, air contained identical proportions of different gases. But until the middle of the eighteenth century, few except hunters and those seeking crystals and gold dared venture high onto mountains: dragons were a proven fact, and superstitions like the spirit of Pontius Pilate kept most people in the valleys or lower hills and passes.

Men must have dreamed of flying from the earliest times, as they watched the effortless soaring of hawks and eagles and longed to be high above the earth, free in the endless oceans of the sky. In 3000 B.C. the Chinese Emperor Shun is said to have been taught to fly by two daughters of another emperor, but the secret must have been well kept. One of the kings of ancient Persia, as legend has it, harnessed wild eagles to his throne, stimulating their flight by holding fish before them. He traveled far and wide before the eagles tired, dropping him in China. There are many variations of the story of how Daedalus, architect of the Labyrinth that housed the Minotaur, escaped from Crete by fashioning wings of wax in which were set real feathers. His son Icarus, intoxicated with freedom, flew too near the sun, which melted the wax, plunging him into the sea, while the more conservative Daedalus landed safely.

But the first authentic aeronautical engineer of whom we have knowledge was Leonardo da Vinci, whose insatiable curiosity and immense genius led him into so many fields of art and science in the fifteenth century. He designed and built a helicopter and a parachute, but most of his passion for flight was directed toward copying birds' wings, and his notebooks contain sketches of different kinds of "ornithopters" — though none flew. He is said to have understood and designed a hot-air balloon. His notebooks were hidden after his death and lost for two centuries, until Napoleon found them and had them published. By that time others had far outstripped Leonardo's efforts.

An imaginative step upward was taken by a distinguished Jesuit scientist and professor of mathematics, Francesco de Lana-Terzi, who, learning of the observations of Torricelli, designed an aerial ship to be lifted by four large globes made of thinnest copper and evacuated like the famous Magdeburg Spheres of Guericke. Lana-Terzi thought that the evacuated spheres would be lighter than air and thus might have considerable lifting power. He visualized large airships carried aloft by the vacuums they contained. But alas, the thin copper spheres were crushed by atmospheric pressure while being evacuated, and the project failed. Later the Jesuit prophetically saw a greater problem: God would surely never allow such a machine to be successful, since it would cause much disturbance among the civil and political governments of mankind.

In 1686 one of the early pioneers in aviation, Laurenco de Guzmao, petitioned the king of Portugal for a patent on an extraordinary airship which he called the "Passarola." Just how this large craft was to fly is not clear; he may already have recognized the lifting power of hot air, but at any rate nothing further seems to have come of it. He did demonstrate that hot air would serve for levitation on August 8, 1709, when he filled a small globe with hot air from the "combustion of various quintessences" and flew it in one of the larger rooms of the king of Portugal's palace. The little model rose to the ceiling, bounced against the wall, and set fire to the draperies. His majesty "was good enough not to take it ill." Apparently Guzmao made no further experiments; there was talk of sorcery and he went to Toledo, where he died in 1724 unhonored and unknown.

Attention then turned to wings, though only briefly, sometimes in the form of gliders, sometimes mechanically operated. In 1755, stimulated no doubt by recent demonstrations that air grew thinner and lighter the higher one went, a Dominican friar named Joseph Galien published specifications for a giant airship, ten times as large as Noah's ark, which would be filled

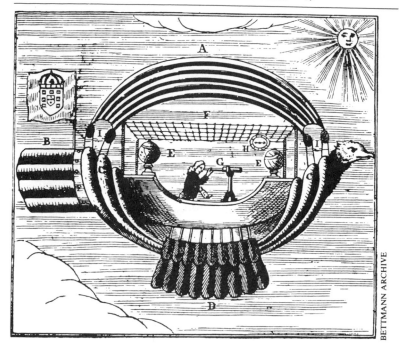

FIGURE 10. WOULD THIS "AIRSHIP" REALLY FLY?

Laurenco de Guzmao demonstrated the lifting power of hot air by flying tiny balloons for the king of Portugal in 1709. But before then he (and doubtless many others long forgotten) dreamed of ships that would "sail the purple twilight" as they did the ocean. Of these the best known is his "Passarola," which, to the best of our knowledge, never existed save on paper. Unable to find for his larger balloons fabric capable of containing a large volume of hot air for long, Guzmao abandoned his dream, leaving to the Montgolfier brothers the fame of first flight. More than a hundred years before Guzmao, Leonardo da Vinci had designed and built models of heavier-than-air machines, but his notebooks were hidden for centuries. Not until the invention of an engine more powerful than man could flight in such a machine become reality.

with thin high-altitude air, but not much progress seems to have been made! Then chemist Joseph Black heard of Henry Cavendish's production of hydrogen and recognized that this gas, so much lighter than air, if suitably enclosed could lift weights. He planned to fill the birth sacs of sheep with hydrogen to demonstrate its lift to his students, but he was diverted and left the actual experiments to an Italian, Tiberias Cavallo, who tried various types of bladders of cloth and paper, none of which was sufficiently tight to contain the hydrogen. Cavallo abandoned the attempt in 1782, after blowing soap bubbles with hydrogen and writing: "In short, soap-balls inflated with inflammable air were the only things of this sort that would ascend into the atmosphere; but as they are very brittle and altogether untractable, they do not seem applicable to any philosophical purpose."

Joseph Montgolfier and his brother Étienne are the most famous of the early pioneers in ballooning. They studied the 1776 edition of Priestley's *Experiments and Observations on Different Kinds of Air* and also began to speculate about the nature of the atmosphere. Joseph, as history has it, was watching bits of paper rising from the fire in his fireplace when he was suddenly struck by the nature of the force that took the light bits — along with smoke — up the chimney. If paper and smoke could rise, why could he not capture the "gas" that propelled them? Why should he not "enclose a cloud in a bag and let the latter be lifted up by the buoyancy of the former"? At first he and Étienne believed that "burned" air was lighter in accordance with the phlogiston theory; smoke was "burned air" and thus had "levity." Only later did they realize that it was heat which provided the lift.

In November 1782 the Montgolfier brothers filled a small taffeta balloon with hot air and, in the greatest secrecy, allowed it to float to the ceiling of a room; shortly afterwards in the open a 750-cubic-foot balloon rose over 600 feet. In these early designs a grill was hung below the narrow open throat of the balloon; on it smouldered a pile of moldy hay (wisdom of the day indicating this was the best fuel) so that the hot smoke rose into the balloon, providing the lift. After many private experiments, on June 4, 1783, the Montgolfiers held a public demonstration before a large and enthusiastic crowd. Their linen balloon was thirty-eight feet in diameter, and after being filled with smoke (and of course hot air), it slowly rose out of sight, carrying 500 pounds, later landing a mile and a half away. Though the brothers still attributed the lift to some substance formed by burning a special kind of hay, Cavallo did understand that hot air was lighter than cold and thus would rise.

There was so much enthusiasm for these early flights that public subscriptions were raised to make more and larger balloons, and in September 1783 a huge balloon was demonstrated before King Louis XVI, his queen, and innumerable people of every rank and age. To dramatize the safety of the flight, live animals were taken up in the basket, which rose over 1,500 feet to the surprise and excitement of the crowd. Though the sheep kicked the rooster, neither was harmed by altitude.

Obviously a man would be next to go — but who? Hearing that a criminal condemned to death had been chosen, an apothecary, Pilâtre de Rozier, insisted that such an honor should not go to the dregs of society and persuaded the Montgolfiers to give him the place. On October 15, 1783, Rozier entered the basket, the fire was stirred, and the balloon rose easily to the end of its tether before being pulled back to earth. A few weeks later a balloon carrying Rozier and a certain Marquis d'Arlandes was allowed to rise free. The two were carried up more than 3,000 feet, landing safely a half hour later several miles away. Men were airborne for the first time!

While all of this was going on, a prominent physicist, Jacques Charles, was developing another form of lift. He had no idea what force had lifted the Montgolfier balloons, but from their dimensions he calculated that the lift could not be as great as that created by the new "inflammable gas" that Henry Cavendish had made by treating iron filings with sulfuric acid.

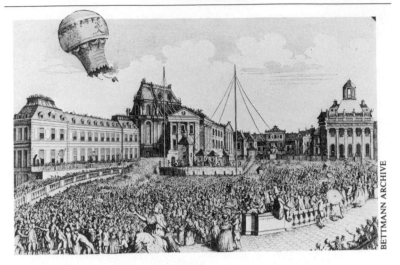

BETTMANN ARCHIVE

FIGURE 11. THE FIRST FREE BALLOON FLIGHT—1783

As Gibbs-Smith wrote:

It came as a great surprise that floating, rather than flapping, flight should first take human beings into the air, especially after the expenditure of so much time and energy by the "tower jumpers" and the breaking of so many bones.

Guzmao had shown that hot air had lifting power, and Black had realized the possibilities of using Cavendish's newly discovered hydrogen in 1767, but did not pursue the matter as Cavallo did a few years later. So it was left to the Montgolfier brothers to first make real man's dream of flight. Their first effort was made indoors in 1782. Their second, more ambitious flight "filled the assembled multitude with silent astonishment which ended with loud unfettered acclamations." They did not know exactly why their balloon rose, supposing it to be due to a special light vapor formed from moldy hay. The Montgolfier brothers lit a fuse that set off an explosion of interest in "aerostation," though they themselves soon abandoned ballooning.

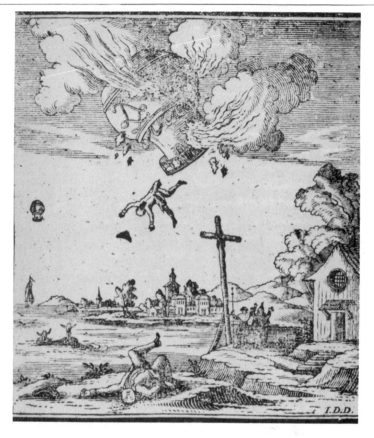

FIGURE 12. BALLOONS CREATED SPECIAL PROBLEMS

For Rozier's first flight the balloon was safely tethered, but after several free flights he became more ambitious. Despite warnings, he filled a balloon with hydrogen and tried to add the lifting power of hot air. The fire below the balloon ignited the hydrogen, and in a spectacular explosion this pioneer aeronaut was killed before a large crowd, including his fiancée.

Since it was difficult to warn rural folks of approaching balloons, it was suggested that flights be preceded by announcers on land and in the air to quiet the fears of the populace. A century or so later, the law required that early automobiles be preceded by a man waving a red flag.

Charles engaged two brothers, Nicolas and Charles Robert, to make a small globe of silk varnished with rubber. On August 23, 1783, this trial balloon was ready, but it took three days to generate enough hydrogen to fill it. Finally, before an immense crowd on August 27, a gun was fired and the balloon rose easily, disappeared into a low cloud, and two hours later landed fifteen miles away, thoroughly startling the people of a tiny village despite a public warning previously issued by the government. The great lifting power of hydrogen had been proven.

Three months later Jacques Charles and Nicolas Robert inflated another balloon, this one twenty-seven feet in diameter, with hydrogen, and (again before a huge crowd) climbed into the basket and took off, waving small flags to show that they were well. They flew much higher and landed twenty-seven miles away, where Nicolas Robert got out while Jacques Charles rose again, more rapidly this time, later writing:

In twenty minutes I was 10,000 feet high, out of sight of terrestrial objects. . . . I passed from the warmth of spring to the cold of winter, a sharp dry cold but not too much to be borne. . . .

In the midst of my delight I felt a violent pain in my right ear and jaw which I ascribed to the dilatation of the air in the cellular construction of these organs.

Jacques Charles was a scientist; we know him best for his gas law, which states that if the pressure on a confined gas is constant, its volume is directly proportional to its temperature.

Ballooning became the current fashion and all sorts of stunts were tried: a certain Mr. Testu-Brissey made an ascent riding on a horse; an opera singer floated above Paris singing arias; and Dr. Leullier-Ducag advocated balloon flights to treat pestilential or nervous fevers, scurvy, hysteria, chlorosis, and melancholy because the air was purer at great heights. A more serious excursion was the crossing of the English Channel by Jean Pierre Blanchard and an American physician, Dr. John Jeffries, who collected samples of air during the flight, and

showed that the composition of all samples, even from different altitudes, was the same. Rozier, rising to the competition,
developed a balloon that combined the lift of heated air and
hydrogen despite the warnings of Jacques Charles that hydrogen was highly flammable. Rozier took off, and the predictable
explosion took place, killing him and his passenger.

Soon the balloonists were competing to make the longest or
the highest flights, and as they went higher into the thin cold
air, the effects of altitude became more and more serious.
Blanchard, whose Channel crossing had brought him notoriety, claimed to have gone up to 32,000 feet, where he "grew
languid [and] felt a numbness, prelude to a dangerous sleep."
His claim was disputed and of course could not be proven,
and he died poor and obscure. Others also claimed altitude records, most credibly a prominent physicist, Joseph Louis Gay-
Lussac, who noted at 22,000 feet that his

*. . . respiration was noticeably hampered; but I was still far from ex-
periencing such severe discomfort as to wish to descend. My pulse and
respiratory rate were much accelerated; and so, breathing very frequently in a very dry air I was not surprised to find my throat so dry
that it was painful to swallow bread. . . . These are all the inconven-
iences I experienced.*

The altitude that could be reached by Montgolfier hot-air
balloons was limited, as was the duration of flight, by the
amount of fuel (usually straw) that could be carried and also
by the decreased combustion in rarefied air, so these enjoyed
limited popularity as hydrogen became more available. Even
the Charlière hydrogen balloons had limitations: ascent and
descent were constantly affected by air temperature, progress
was deranged by wind, and since no replacement hydrogen
could be carried, once it had been vented through the special
escape valve, further ascent was possible only by dropping off
weights — usually sand — which experienced aeronauts threw
out in small handfuls with the cunning of a miser. After his famous Channel crossing, Jeffries reported that only discarding

five or six pounds of urine had saved him and Blanchard from a dunking!

By the end of the century attention turned to heavier-than-air machines. George Cayley published important articles on the history and principles of aerial navigation, and Walker wrote a *Treatise on the Art of Flying by Mechanical Means* in 1810 that is remarkable in its perceptions. But without a light-weight engine, such machines were not practicable and interest turned back to ballooning.

An English meteorologist, Henry Coxwell, and James Glaisher were carried very high, possibly to 29,000 feet, in a hydrogen balloon in 1862 and escaped death from hypoxia only because Coxwell, in his last conscious moments, was able to pull the release valve with his teeth, releasing hydrogen and allowing the balloon to descend. Glaisher became something of an authority on the effects of high altitude and after a great many ascents felt that he had developed a tolerance:

At length I became so acclimatized to the effects of a more rarefied atmosphere, that I could breathe at an elevation of four miles at least above the earth without inconvenience, and I have no doubt that this faculty of acclimatization might be so developed as to have a very important bearing upon the philosophical uses of balloon ascents.

By then it was almost a century since the vital properties of oxygen had been described, and even longer since Mayow and others had shown that small animals died when deprived of it in a closed vessel. The decrease in barometric pressure at altitude had been demonstrated, along with the attendant decrease in oxygen pressure. Yet the early balloonists had not fully grasped that the dangers of altitude were due to lack of oxygen and could be prevented by breathing that gas. It remained for an extraordinary man, often called the father of altitude physiology, to show how the catastrophes could be prevented.

Paul Bert was born in Burgundy less than a hundred miles from Paris. He first studied engineering, later changed to law, which he found too boring, then entered medicine, graduating at the age of thirty, though he never practiced medicine. Instead he studied under the great physiologist Claude Bernard and found his true love in experimental physiology, including transplant surgery. For almost twenty years he studied the effects of reduced and increased pressure on small animals and later on man, using steel cylinders (or bells) specially designed for his laboratory. His experiments clearly showed that breathing air under reduced pressure — as at altitude — was dangerous because of oxygen lack, and that breathing oxygen, even under considerably reduced pressure, restored normal function. Bert turned to the study of blood and was able to define the first crude curves showing the relationships between hemoglobin and oxygen under different pressures, thus laying the foundations for much later work in oxygen transport.

Bert collected accounts from travelers as well as scientists from all over the world and, in addition to his studies in decompression chambers, became interested in the opportunities that balloons offered for studying altitude. In March 1874 two aspiring aeronauts, Joseph Crocé-Spinelli and Theodor Sivel, came to Bert's laboratory "with the purpose of studying upon themselves the disagreeable effects of decompression and the favorable influence of superoxygenated air" in preparation for an attempt to set a new altitude record. During the hour they spent in the chamber the pressure was reduced to that equivalent to 24,000 feet, and they experienced dimming of vision, dulling of mind, and difficulty with calculations, all promptly relieved by a few inhalations of oxygen, which they breathed whenever the symptoms became severe. Crocé-Spinelli had already been up to 15,000 feet in a balloon without noticing any unpleasant effects and may have been a bit blasé about the risks. Bert, in contrast, was very much concerned and wanted to demonstrate conclusively how effectively oxygen could protect the balloonists. On March 28 he had himself decompressed in the chamber to 21,000 feet, breathing oxygen without interruption from 16,000 feet up. From the hour-and-a-half experiment he concluded "that continuous inhalations of oxygen,

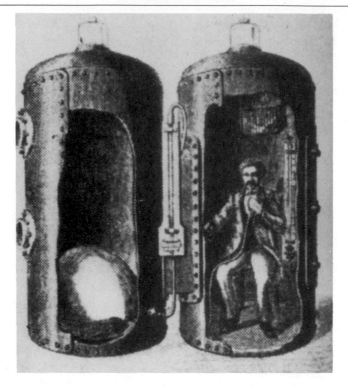

FIGURE 13. PAUL BERT'S DECOMPRESSION CHAMBER

Paul Bert used this steel "bell" or decompression chamber, given him by his generous sponsor Dr. Jourdannet, for studying the effects of high altitude in the laboratory. He was able to evacuate the chamber to simulate any desired altitude, and in it one person at a time could experience lack of oxygen while protected by outside observers. This was before the days of pressurized gas cylinders, but by keeping a leather sac filled with oxygen in an adjoining chamber (connected by a small pipe to the subject's chamber), Bert could supply oxygen or allow the subject to breathe the thinner air. This showed dramatically how beneficial oxygen was at altitude, after showing how much the mind and body deteriorated while breathing only air. The lesson undoubtedly saved many lives, though the *Zenith*'s crew did not take enough oxygen to prevent the death of two of the three. Bert also used the "bell" to study the effects of increased pressure, as for example on divers.

after having checked painful symptoms, will prevent them from reappearing, though the barometric pressure continues to fall."

On March 22, 1874, Crocé-Spinelli and Sivel ascended to approximately 24,000 feet (7,300 meters) in a great balloon, "The Polar Star," and wrote:

We felt in our flight impressions similar to those which we had experienced in the decompression bells of M. Bert in which several days before we were taken to a pressure of 304 mm* (23,000 feet). . . . In the bell, the pure oxygen which we were breathing caused dizzy spells like those of drunkenness, whereas on the contrary we were very comfortable with the two mixtures, one of 40% oxygen and 60% nitrogen, and the other of 70% oxygen and 30% nitrogen which M. Bert had furnished for our ascent. . . .

After these experiments Bert and the balloonists were fully convinced of

. . . the favorable effects of inhalation of oxygen. Return of strength and appetite, decrease of headache, restoration of clear vision, calmness of mind, all the phenomena already observed in the cylinders of the laboratory . . . we produced with a certainty . . . that was very striking.

Consequently they arranged to carry oxygen in three large leather bags on their record-breaking flight. Bert was in Paris on the day planned for the attempt. Crocé-Spinelli had written to him that they would have approximately 150 liters of oxygen in the three skin bags. Bert was alarmed. He wrote back immediately: "In the lofty elevations where this artificial respiration will be indispensable to you, for three men you should count on a consumption of at least 20 liters per minute; see how soon your supply will be exhausted."

But the letter arrived too late. The story of the flight of the

---

* Scientists were beginning to define altitude by the barometric pressure, usually measured in the height of the column of mercury in a barometer, normal sea level pressure sustaining the column at 760 mm. One torr = one mm mercury.

balloon *Zenith* on April 15, 1875, is dramatic, but it is only one of the many tragedies that occurred as daring men used balloons and later heavier-than-air machines to reach great altitudes without thorough understanding of the risks of oxygen lack. Bert quotes the vivid account, given immediately after the flight, by the sole survivor, Gaston Tissandier, in which he describes in detail the symptoms of hypoxia, which overcame him somewhere above 25,000 feet and would have killed him as well as his two companions had he not somehow gathered strength and will to vent some hydrogen and cause the *Zenith* to descend:

The last very clear memory that remains to me of the ascent goes back to a moment a little before this. . . . Soon I was keeping absolutely motionless, without suspecting that perhaps I had already lost use of my movements. . . . Towards 7,500 m the numbness one experiences is extraordinary. The body and mind weaken little by little, gradually, unconsciously and without one's knowledge. One does not suffer at all, quite the contrary. One experiences an inner joy, as if it were an effect of the inundating flood of light. One becomes indifferent; one no longer thinks of the perilous situation or the danger; one rises and is happy to rise. . . . I soon felt so weak that I could not even turn my head to look at my companions. . . . I wanted to seize the oxygen tube but could not raise my arm. My mind, however, was still very lucid. I was still looking at the barometer, my eyes were fixed on the needle which soon reached the pressure number of 290, then 280, beyond which it passed. . . . I wanted to cry out "We are at 8,000 meters," but my tongue was paralyzed. Suddenly I closed my eyes and fell inert, entirely losing consciousness.

This tragedy was neither the first nor last caused by lack of oxygen in man's odyssey toward the heavens. Coxwell and Tissandier were fortunate and unusual. As we will see, hypoxia is so subtle, so insidious, that its victim is often incapable of saving himself before he is aware of the danger, and death soon follows. Looking back on these pioneer balloonists, whether we think them heroic or foolhardy, we marvel at their courage.

Knowing what we know today, it's difficult to believe that some reached anywhere near the altitudes they claimed. No matter, they were surely as brave as those who sailed off into the unknown oceans or who rode our early rockets into space, and they gave us a legacy of great value.

Paul Bert seems to have lost some of his enthusiasm for altitude studies after the *Zenith* accident, and he became more active in politics. He was appointed Resident General in Indo-China to resolve the endless turmoil there, but like so many thousands in the century to come, he was unsuccessful and died at age fifty-three, five months after his arrival. His lasting monument is his book *La Pression Barométrique,* a huge collection of all that he could learn from others and from his own extensive studies of barometric pressure and altitude physiology. Though little known for some decades, the French text was translated into English in 1943 by Dr. and Mrs. Fred Hitchcock at Ohio State University and has served as an inspiration and stimulus to all who study space, the atmosphere, and mountains.

Bert had been encouraged throughout his career by a wealthy patron, Dr. Denis Jourdannet, who had become interested in altitude during his travels in Mexico. Jourdannet generously gave him much of the equipment and the steel decompression chambers which a Dr. Junod in 1835 was the first to use.

Bert was strongly influenced by another physician, also ahead of his time: Dr. Conrad Meyer-Ahrens of Leipzig, who had, in 1854, published a book containing a summary of his conclusions from many travelers' tales and many experiments:

The principal symptoms (of altitude illness) or at least those which occur oftenest in man are: discomfort, distaste for food, especially distaste for wine (however, the contrary has sometimes been noted), intense thirst (especially for water, which quenches the thirst best), nausea, vomiting; accelerated and panting respiration; dyspnea, acceleration of the pulse, throbbing of the large arteries and the temples;

violent palpitations, oppression, anxiety, asphyxia; vertigo, headache, tendency to syncope, unconquerable desire for sleep, though the sleep does not refresh but is disturbed by anguish; finally, astonishing and very strange muscular fatigue. These symptoms do not always appear all together. . . . Others are observed, although less frequently, such as pulmonary, renal, and intestinal hemorrhages (in animals also); vomiting of blood; oozing of blood from the mucous membrane of the lips and the skin (due merely to the desiccation of these membranes), blunting of sensory perceptions and the intelligence, impatience, irritability . . . finally, buzzing in the ears. . . . All that we have just said about the etiology of mountain sickness shows (1) that it appears at varying altitudes; (2) that meteorological conditions, temporary or general personal characteristics, and the speed of walking vary the altitude at which one is attacked and the severity and number of the symptoms. . . . In my opinion, the principal role belongs to the decrease of the absolute quantity of oxygen in the rarefied air, the rapidity of evaporation and the intense action of light, direct or reflected from snow, whereas the direct action of the decreased pressure should be placed in the second rank. I find the immediate causes of mountain sickness in the changes made in the composition and formation of the blood by the decrease in oxygen and the exaggerated evaporation, changes to which are added others due to the action of light on the cerebral function, an action which affects the preparation of the blood liquid.

We cannot improve much on this today!

Balloons were widely used for recreation, for excitement, and (in our Civil War and the Franco-Prussian War of 1870) for important military missions, as well as for research, but as the century ended it was clear that heavier-than-air machines would soon fly, and the Age of Aviation began. The first tentative flights scarcely threatened lack of oxygen, but the advent of World War I confirmed that high-flying aircraft would become decisive factors in warfare. Within a few short years engines and airframes were able to go higher than could pilots unaided by oxygen, and fighting took place higher and higher, with all its terror, just as Lana-Terzi and da Vinci had predicted. Altitude physiology received a tremendous stimulus from war high in the atmosphere, and by the nineteen twenties sophisticated studies were again being done on high mountains, because aircraft went up too fast and for too short a time for the kind of work which needed to be done.

Both in war and peace, lack of oxygen at altitude has killed many because of bravado, or ignorance, or, more often, because their oxygen equipment failed. But hypoxia in aviation is quite different from that on mountains or in most illnesses: it is more abrupt in onset, more severe, and the outcome more dangerous. The story of oxygen in aviation is a dramatic one but not relevant to this book, which deals with more gradual, subtler, and far more common problems.

As the nineteenth century ended, most scientists were in agreement that the basic cause of altitude illness was lack of oxygen due to decreased barometric pressure. One exception was a distinguished mountaineering physiologist, Angelo Mosso, who extended his laboratory studies to the summit of Monte Rosa (15,025 feet) on the Swiss-Italian frontier, where Queen Margherita of Italy sponsored and dedicated in person a small stone laboratory. Not many queens would have made the long and not always easy climb, even unimpeded by the long skirts and numerous ladies-in-waiting mandated by those times.

Mosso published his observations in a fascinating book, *Life of Man on the High Alps,* in 1896, which was translated into English two years later. He concluded that lack of oxygen could not adequately explain all that happened at altitude, and coined the word *acapnia,* meaning lack of carbon dioxide, which he thought would cause the symptoms. There was — and still is — some truth in this because the strong stimulus to breathe more than normally does wash out carbon dioxide from lungs and blood at altitude, and the result is a drift toward the alkaline side, which does cause problems. But Mosso's ideas did not gain much acceptance, and Bert, and later Haldane and Barcroft, conclusively showed that lack of oxygen was the primary but (as we will see later) not the sole cause of altitude problems.

Mosso has left us several major contributions, however. First, he observed irregular breathing at altitude during sleep, attributing this correctly to derangement of the normal stimuli to breathing and suggesting that this was why mountain sickness was worse at night or early in the morning. He also wondered what was happening in the brain to cause the headache so characteristic of mountain sickness, and to study this he was able to find two youths who had holes in their skulls as a result of accidents. The first (Cesar Lasagno) was taken in Mosso's decompression chamber to about 17,000 feet, where there was "some diminution in the tonicity of the blood vessels of the brain" but no evidence of congestion or anemia. The second boy (Emmanuele Favre) was given a mixture of 10 percent oxygen in nitrogen to breathe, equivalent to breathing air at 18,000 feet. He had some minor symptoms which Mosso attributed to "a disturbance in nutrition of the brain" rather than to "paralysis of the blood vessels." Mosso did not observe any swelling, but did conclude, correctly, that altitude headache was somehow related to circulation.

His third contribution was to record for the first time details of the death of a young physician high on Mont Blanc, the first record we have of high-altitude pulmonary edema.

As our century began, balloons had taken men more than five miles above the earth, briefly and occasionally tragically. Adventurous mountaineers had reached 21,000 feet, but many had been miserably sick and some had died. The use of decompression chambers had shown that decreased pressure led to all the signs and symptoms seen at altitude — and when these were prevented or relieved by breathing oxygen, it seemed obvious that lack of oxygen due to the decreased barometric pressure was the basic cause of altitude sickness. Other causes — some outlandish, but some at least partly correct — had been proposed. Powered aircraft had already begun to bring great opportunities as well as risks and grave threats to mankind. Three centuries earlier, who at that time would have believed men would be able to sample air using helium balloons thirty miles above earth, walk on the moon, and control rockets sent millions of miles into space? Mt. Everest had been discovered and its height measured, but no one then believed it could be climbed, let alone without oxygen.

Chapter Four

MOVING AIR: RESPIRATION

OF ALL THE STUFFS essential to life, only oxygen is neither manufactured nor stored in our bodies: the supply must be replenished almost as rapidly as it is used. This places severe limits on where we — like most mammals — can go and what we can do. Unlike the turtle, man cannot spend a long, cold winter snugly buried in mud at the bottom of a pond. Nor can we hibernate like bears or ground squirrels. We cannot even stay underwater for an hour like whales and seals. We must breathe to live — and we must take in as much oxygen as we consume, and as fast as we consume it.

When John Mayow watched his mouse die beneath the bell jar he concluded that life depended on "a vital spirit . . . that is by means of respiration transmitted into the mass of the blood and the fermentation and the heating of the blood are produced by it."

Scheele, Boyle, Hooke, and finally Priestley and Lavoisier repeated such experiments many times before it became clear that all animals must have this "vital spirit" to "burn" foodstuffs that fuel every activity, much as a candle must have air in order to burn. Everything we do — thinking or dreaming, running or climbing mountains, eating, getting angry or making love — all require oxygen to release the energy that pumps the blood, moves the muscles, secretes the hormones, and excretes the wastes.

Some functions can continue for a few minutes without oxygen (anaerobically), but only by accumulating an oxygen debt which is very short term and must be repaid, with interest. We do have a small reserve or storehouse in a special form of blood pigment in muscles called myoglobin, which holds some oxygen in the larger muscles for quick release when there's demand for more oxygen than blood can deliver rapidly. But the human body is strictly dependent on an uninterrupted supply of oxygen — greater during work, less during rest.

To maintain such a steady supply, we rely on what is called the oxygen transport system. This is a short way of describing the process of acquisition, transportation, delivery, and utilization of oxygen. Acquisition takes place when we breathe, as the lungs fill with air from which oxygen will diffuse into the blood. Transportation is accomplished by the flowing blood in which oxygen is loosely combined with the red pigment called hemoglobin. Delivery occurs when the large blood vessels, dividing into ever smaller ones, finally become capillaries barely large enough for the red cells to tumble through, where oxygen diffuses from the blood into the fluid-filled tissue around our living cells. And utilization — for which the whole system is organized — takes place in tiny parts (mitochondria) in each cell. There oxygen is used to release energy, which takes many forms depending on the type of cell.

Less noticed, but just as important, is passage of the waste product carbon dioxide in the opposite direction — from cells to lungs to outside air, which also makes possible rapid adjustment of the acidity of blood and tissues. If blood becomes too acid, we breathe more deeply or faster to eliminate carbon dioxide, which, dissolved in water, is a weak acid. Or, should we err on the alkaline side, breathing tends to slow, and we hold back this weak acid. Other waste products are also carried from cells to lungs or liver or kidney, where they are eliminated in one way or another.

The oxygen transport system is beautifully suited to its task. It is flexible and can double or triple its capacity at each stage, being swiftly responsive to many feedback loops. It is specialized to carry oxygen and carbon dioxide, unless interfered with by an improbable alien like carbon monoxide or cyanide. It has multiple checks and balances and redundant control points which function so smoothly we are seldom aware of them. And it is multi-purposed: the whole system helps maintain a constant body temperature, stable acidity, and a suitable level of hydration. Blood carries free passengers such as hormones (messenger substances) and enzymes (catalysts), as well as normal and unnatural wastes like alcohol, drugs, and many other unwanted materials.

As we try to understand man's response to altitude, we need to look at each part of the system: acquisition, transportation, delivery, and utilization. It is an enormously complex system with more circuits than the largest computer. Before examining each stage, it will be helpful to understand another shorthand term: the "oxygen cascade."

Remember that John Dalton described partial pressure as the pressure any gas in a mixture of gases would exert if it were the only gas occupying the same enclosed space. This enables us to talk of "oxygen partial pressure" and "partial pressure of carbon dioxide" and to use these in mathematical equations. We can think of oxygen as having "high" pressure in outside air, lower pressure in the lungs where it is diluted with carbon dioxide and water vapor, and still lower pressure by the time it has reached the cells. This drop in (partial) pressure is the oxygen cascade. At each stage in the transport system, some pressure is lost. And it is by minimizing the loss at each stage that man is able to live and work at altitudes (or in environments) where the oxygen pressure is low.

Air everywhere on earth is made up of 20.96 percent oxygen and almost 80 percent nitrogen with traces of other gases. By Dalton's law we easily calculate that the partial pressure of oxygen in air at sea level (barometric pressure 760 torr) is about 21 percent of 760, or 160 torr. At 18,000 feet, where barometric pressure is half that at sea level, oxygen partial pressure is 21 percent of 380, or about 80 torr.

When we breathe in, the entering air mixes with the outgoing and picks up water vapor, which — like any other gas — has a partial pressure. This is 47 torr at body temperature, because air is probably fully saturated in the body. The carbon dioxide and water vapor deep in the lungs reduce the pressure of oxygen there to about 100–110 torr, and this is the first "drop" in the oxygen cascade. We decrease this drop by breathing faster and/or more deeply.

Once in the innermost parts of the lungs, oxygen must pass through two membranes to enter the red cells, by a process called diffusion, and this causes another small drop in pressure, the second in the cascade.

Safely attached to hemoglobin, oxygen is carried throughout the body with no further drop until it must leave its carrier and diffuse again, from blood into tissues, and from tissues into cells. Here there is a further small drop in pressure, down the cascade.

Finally oxygen enters each cell and becomes available to fuel the complex energy cycles run by the mitochondria, and in this process the final pressure drop — probably to zero — occurs. The cascade has reached bottom.

Understanding the oxygen cascade is important because it is by altering one or many of these "drops" that man (and many other mammals) can survive moderate oxygen lack.

With this introduction, let's look at the stages, starting with breathing in and out, inhalation and exhalation, usually called respiration or ventilation.

The chest cavity is separated from the abdominal cavity by a great platelike muscle, the diaphragm; the chest contains heart and vessels (slung in a thin tough sac) and the lungs, which open to the outside air through bronchial tubes, trachea, mouth, and nose. Expansion of the chest is accomplished by small muscles between the ribs, and by flattening of the dia-

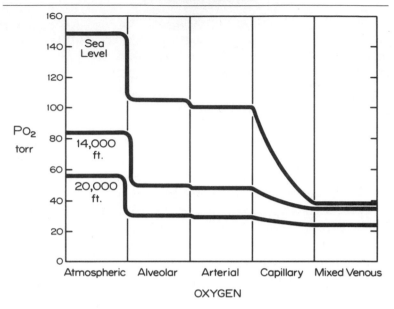

FIGURE 14. THE OXYGEN CASCADE

At each stage in its passage from outside air to tissues, oxygen loses some pressure. This series of drops is known as the oxygen cascade. At each stage some measures will minimize the drop, thereby raising the oxygen available to tissues, just as at each stage there are diseases or abnormalities that can increase the drop, thereby decreasing the tissue oxygenation.

Between outside air and alveolar air, oxygen pressure falls sharply because mixing is incomplete. Overbreathing improves mixing and decreases this drop.

Between alveolar air and lung capillary blood (which will be fully oxygenated as it leaves the lung), there is a small oxygen pressure drop due to resistance of the alveolar-capillary membranes. This may increase sharply due to chronic disease like fibrosis, or acute disease like early pulmonary edema. This "A-a gradient" can be quite important in oxygen delivery.

Little if any oxygen pressure is lost during transit of blood from lungs to tissue capillaries.

As oxygen diffuses from capillary into individual cells, more pressure is lost due to membrane resistance and to the distance between capillary and cell. By opening up new capillaries, this capillary-cell gradient can be decreased, whereas accumulation of water in the tissues or sluggish blood flow will increase the gradient, aggravating tissue oxygen lack.

MOVING AIR: RESPIRATION *71*

Mixed venous blood is the blood entering the right side of the heart from all veins of the body and is an indicator of both the body's need for oxygen and its utilization of oxygen. Mixed venous oxygen falls as exertion increases; mixed venous is lower at altitude than at sea level. It is a better indicator of tissue oxygenation than arterial blood oxygen.

---

phragm, which is normally domed. As the rib cage expands, the chest cavity enlarges like a bellows, allowing atmospheric pressure to push the outside air in. When the chest contracts, the diaphragm relaxes and staler air is driven out.

One cannot improve on the description of breathing in and out written by John Mayow in 1674, on the verge of discovering oxygen a century before Priestley and Lavoisier:

With respect then to the entrance of air into the lungs, I think it is to be maintained that it is caused . . . by the pressure of the atmosphere. For as the air, on account of the weight of the superincumbent atmosphere . . . rushes into all empty places . . . it follows that the air passes through the nostrils and the trachea up to the bronchia. . . . When the inner sides of the thorax . . . are drawn outwards by muscles . . . and the space in the thorax is enlarged, the air which is nearest the bronchio inlets . . . rushes under the full pressure of the atmosphere into the cavities of the lungs. . . . From this we conclude that the lungs are distended by the air rushing in, and that they do not expand of themselves, as some have supposed.

The upper airways — mouth and nose and trachea — provide air conditioning. Their membrane linings are kept moist by diffusion of water from a dense network of small blood vessels just beneath the surface, which also warms the in-rushing air. A thin film of mucus lines the airways, capturing small particles much as flypaper catches flies. The trachea and larger bronchial tubes are also lined with cells that have hairlike appendages — cilia — which constantly sweep the film of mucus and its wastes upward to the mouth to be swallowed or spit out. By the time outside air has moved only a short distance, it is saturated with water, warmed, and cleansed of all but the

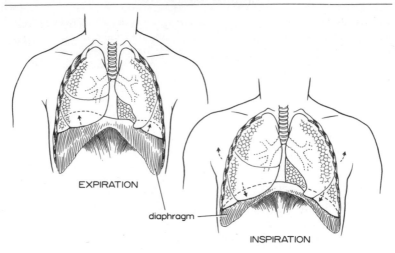

EXPIRATION

diaphragm

INSPIRATION

FIGURE 15. RESPIRATION:
HOW AIR ENTERS AND LEAVES THE LUNGS

Inspiration is an active process, requiring muscular work: the dome-shaped diaphragm contracts and flattens, increasing the vertical dimensions of the chest cavity, and the small muscles between the ribs also contract, pulling the ribs outward and upward, thus increasing the dimensions fore and aft. As a result, just as Mayow perceived, air is pushed into the increased space by outside atmospheric pressure. Expiration, by contrast, is more passive: the diaphragm relaxes and returns to its upward dome shape. The intercostal muscles also relax and the rib cage becomes smaller. Air then is under more pressure than outside the chest and flows out. One result of living for generations at altitude is enlargement of the chest.

smallest particles. Even when the rush of air is ten or twenty times greater than normal during strenuous exertion, air conditioning is complete. This means that the body loses a great deal of water and heat when we breathe the cold, dry air of altitude; this is not recaptured during expiration, and so breathing dry air results in loss of a great volume of body water, terribly important to mountain climbers.

Cold air must be warmed to body temperature as it is

breathed in, and consequently heat is lost with each exhalation. When breathing is very rapid, obviously more heat will be lost. Sir Brian Matthews pointed out years ago that evaporation of water from the mucous membranes that line the nose, mouth, and the bronchial tree also soaks up heat, and calculated that near the top of Everest a man may lose more heat evaporating moisture to saturate the bone-dry air than he can replace by "burning" his food and by working.

The trachea divides into major bronchi, which in turn divide into smaller and smaller bronchi and these into bronchioles. Each of these small tubes ends in a cluster of tiny air sacs 0.25 mm in diameter, called alveoli (from the Latin for "concave vessel"), which is where exchange of oxygen and carbon dioxide takes place between inspired air and blood. In the normal human lung, each of the 300 million alveoli is enmeshed in a network of small capillary blood vessels, terminations of the branching vessels which carry blood from all over the body, through the heart and into the lungs. After passing the alveoli, these capillaries join again, like brooks into streams and rivers, to form the large vessels which return blood filled with oxygen and depleted of carbon dioxide to the heart and thence to all parts of the body.

A crucial step in respiration occurs during the brief moments when blood is in these capillaries, for it is only there that oxygen and carbon dioxide can pass between alveoli and blood. The pulmonary capillaries are only slightly larger (and many are slightly smaller) than the diameter of a red blood cell. The tiny disc-shaped red cells are twisted and distorted (and might easily become stuck) as they pass through capillaries, which are thin-walled, fragile, and elastic, each serving several different alveoli. At altitude, and during exertion, more capillaries open, allowing a larger flow of blood to come in contact with the alveoli.

The passage of a gas (in this case oxygen or carbon dioxide) through a semipermeable membrane (the alveolar wall) depends on several factors: among the more important are the

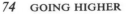

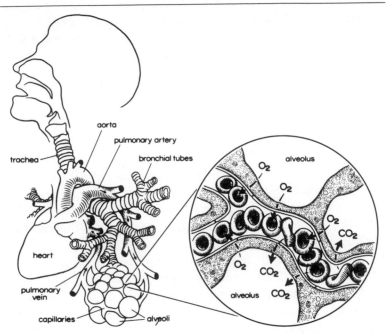

FIGURE 16. THE LUNG CAPILLARIES AND ALVEOLI

The heart and its great vessels (aorta, pulmonary artery, and great veins) are so intimately intertwined with the airways (trachea and bronchial tubes) that they are difficult to show except in a foreshortened illustration such as this. The bronchial tubes branch into ever smaller passages, each terminating in a cluster of air sacs (alveoli) much like a bunch of grapes. With each breath air moves in and out of this intricate system, partially replacing "stale" air in the alveoli with fresher air from outside. Each alveolus (smaller than a pinhead) is surrounded by a network of capillary blood vessels, barely large enough to allow red cells to pass, and each capillary serves several alveoli. Oxygen diffuses from the alveolus (where its pressure is higher) through the alveolar wall, through a narrow space (interstitial space), and through the capillary wall into the red blood cells. Blood arriving in the lungs contains more carbon dioxide than is in the alveoli, so carbon dioxide flows from capillary to alveolus and actually expedites passage of oxygen in the opposite direction. The whole transaction takes only a fraction of a second, but by the time each bit of blood has passed through alveolar capillaries, it has taken on a full load of oxygen and released most of its carbon dioxide. High altitude, where oxygen pressure is lower in the atmosphere and hence in the alveolus, decreases the flow of oxygen into blood but does not affect the release of carbon dioxide. Diseases that impair ventilation or thicken or change the alveolar walls also impair oxygen flow, but they affect carbon dioxide flow as well.

---

difference in pressure of the gas between the two sides of the membrane, the area and thickness of the membrane, and a "diffusion coefficient" peculiar to the gas. Division of the lung into millions of tiny air sacs provides a diffusing area of about 750 square feet — about 100 times as large as the area of a single sac the size of the entire chest cavity. The difference in pressure between the alveolus and the capillary is called the Alveolar-arterial (A-a) gradient.

So large is the alveolar surface area available for diffusion that oxygen diffuses rapidly through the alveolar walls at sea level, where its partial pressure is much higher than that in blood arriving in the lungs. Diffusion is complete in less than half a second at sea level, while a red blood cell takes three fourths of a second or even longer to traverse the capillary adjoining the alveolus. Transit or exposure time is not a limiting factor at sea level, though it may become so at great altitude. The normal A-a gradient in youth is 2 to 5 torr, but it increases to 10 or 15 torr in old age. Usually — but not always — the A-a gradient decreases during exercise, but at altitude it may either increase or decrease depending on changes that we will examine in later chapters.

The A-a oxygen gradient as we measure it reflects the overall difference between alveolar and arterial oxygen pressures — it's an average for all of both lungs. We know now that in different parts of the lung the gradient will be different depending on several important influences. If, for example, there's some local infection like pneumonia, that area may receive less air than normal lung, while its blood flow is normal or even increased. In another case, blood flow may be impeded by any of several causes — small blood clots, for example, or spasm of the small vessels — while ventilation is normal. These are examples of inequity between ventilation and circulation, which we call ventilation–perfusion mismatch. When mismatch exists, it increases the A-a gradient. Mismatch also results when some blood goes through vessels which bypass alveoli, because this blood goes through the lung without being exposed to oxygen. Such shunts occur in many people, but they are usually unimportant; when they do occur they may contribute substantially to altitude illness, particularly high-altitude pulmonary edema (HAPE).

The most common cause of an abnormally large gradient between alveolar and arterial oxygen pressure is chronic lung disease, such as emphysema or fibrosis. In emphysema the walls between alveoli break down and the larger sacs that result have less area through which oxygen can diffuse; in extreme cases the diffusing area may be less than half normal. In cases of fibrosis, the barrier between the alveoli and the capillaries is thickened and diffusion (which depends in part on the thickness of the barrier) is impeded. Often emphysema and fibrosis occur together and the A-a gradient may be very large.

The trachea, bronchi, and alveoli are dead-end passages, and air moves in and out rather than through as it does in some animals. This ebb and flow is called the "tidal air" and is of course increased with deeper or faster breathing. The greater the tidal air, the better the mixing of purer outside air with stale air deep in the lungs. So anything that decreases ventilation interferes with tidal air and is likely to decrease oxygen in the alveoli. A good example is the slow, shallow breathing characteristic of sleep in some persons, which may — especially at high altitude — decrease oxygen in the blood quite significantly. Conversely, overbreathing increases alveolar oxygen, and many climbers practice deliberate overbreathing (sometimes called "grunt breathing"), which was developed as an emergency procedure during World War II for aviators who lost their oxygen supply at altitude.

But just as the partial pressure of oxygen in the alveoli is increased by deeper breathing, so too is the partial pressure of carbon dioxide decreased. Carbon dioxide is constantly formed in tissues as part of combustion, in greater amounts during work. It diffuses rapidly from tissues into blood, where it is carried partly in solution, but mostly in a loose equilibrium as carbonate-bicarbonate. This is a most fortunate arrangement because carbon dioxide diffuses twenty times as rapidly as does oxygen and would tend to rush out of the blood into the lungs too rapidly were it not slowed a little by this loose chemical combination.

Carbon dioxide is the principal regulator of the acidity of the blood, and a very precise one it is, since its level can change in a second or two depending on the level of breathing and the amount of work being done. Overbreathing deliberately may lower carbon dioxide enough to make the blood too alkaline and cause a condition known as hyperventilation syndrome, which causes faintness, tingling in fingers and toes, dizziness, painful cramps, and even collapse. The climber or flyer who deliberately tries to control his breathing at altitude must walk a narrow path between the Scylla of oxygen lack (if he breathes too little) and the Charybdis of carbon dioxide lack (if he breathes too much). It's tricky!

Once oxygen is in the lung capillaries, it enters the red cells swiftly and combines with hemoglobin to be carried to all parts of the body without losing appreciable pressure on the way. In the tissue capillaries, the higher pressure of oxygen in the arterial end of the capillary causes oxygen to "flow downhill" as it were, diffusing through the capillary wall, through the loose (interstitial) space between cells, through the thin cell wall into the watery fluid called cytoplasm that fills each cell, and finally into the minute granules — the mitochondria (from the Latin for "thread-grains") — where the real action is. The flow of oxygen is matched by the flow — in the opposite direction — of carbon dioxide, from cells where it is formed, through various barriers into the venous end of capillaries, and thence to the alveoli and out.

Understanding the oxygen cascade gives us a better idea of where the delivery of oxygen is most affected by going to high altitude: (1) in the lungs, because the partial pressure of oxygen is lower; (2) between lungs and blood, if fluid or foreign material accumulates there; (3) in the blood, if there are not enough red blood cells to carry oxygen; (4) in the capillaries, if there is not enough partial pressure of oxygen to move it from blood to cells; and finally, (5) in the cells, if the mitochondria or the enzyme systems are not maximally efficient. The cascade also suggests where the body may adjust to oxygen lack by certain changes.

It's obvious that we can increase the partial pressure of oxygen in blood most if we improve ventilation of the lungs by deeper breathing, which results in more efficient mixing of fresh air with that deep in the lung. Ventilation is the most important adjustment we can make.

We are seldom conscious of our breathing because it is dictated by stimuli we only dimly perceive. The control of breathing is one of the more fascinating chapters in human physiology — and appropriate breathing is crucial to staying well at altitude.

We know that strenuous exertion, sudden excitement, fear, passion, or even stepping under a cold shower makes us breathe faster or deeper or both, even though there may not, in some cases, be any immediate, obvious demand for more oxygen. We know that during sleep our breathing becomes shallow, often irregular, and consequently our lungs are less well ventilated — an important effect at high altitude. How and where are these changes dictated?

It's obvious that strenuous exertion — or fear-induced preparation for fight or flight — requires more than the normal flow of oxygen. Exertion calls for increased breathing because carbon dioxide or lactic acid accumulates, making the blood more acid, or because stimuli are sent to the brain from the working muscles. Fear is a more subtle stimulus: breathing increases before the demand for oxygen develops. A cold shower

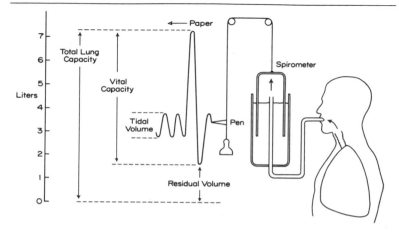

FIGURE 17. DEFINING VENTILATION

After taking in the deepest possible breath, the subject exhales into a bell jar over water (spirometer). Rise and fall of the spirometer are recorded on paper on a revolving drum. Even after the fullest expiration some residual air remains in the lung. Residual air plus the maximum volume that can be exhaled after the maximum inhalation is called total lung capacity. Total lung capacity minus the residual air is the vital capacity, or useful breathing capacity. In normal breathing at rest, inspiration and expiration move a much smaller volume, known as the tidal air. This simple set of measurements is made more informative by measuring the number of seconds it takes to move air, thus obtaining the timed vital capacity. A decrease in vital capacity may be one of the earliest signs of beginning altitude sickness (pulmonary edema); changes in several of these measurements occur in different lung diseases and at altitude.

stimulates the skin nerve endings that direct blood flow and, again in anticipation, call for more breathing. Passion arouses both physical and emotional stimuli to greater effort and greater need for oxygen.

We also know that lack of oxygen stimulates breathing; this is an early and effective response to altitude. It's reasonable to expect that hypoxia would initiate instructions to breathe more deeply. It's also reasonable to expect that when carbon dioxide

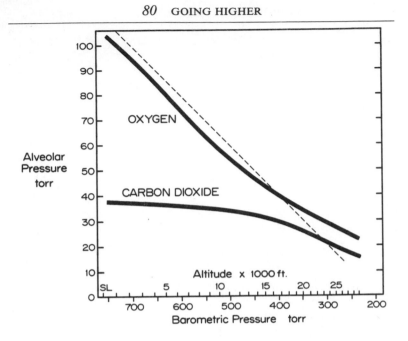

FIGURE 18. CHANGES IN ALVEOLAR GASES AT ALTITUDE

With increasing altitude, the pressure of oxygen in alveolar air decreases, as does that of carbon dioxide. However, around 8,000 feet ventilation increases enough to cause considerable improvement in the mixing of incoming air with that deep in the lungs. As a result oxygen pressure falls less steeply, but carbon dioxide more steeply as the individual goes still higher. The broken line shows how atmospheric pressure (scaled along the bottom of the lower axis) falls as altitude (scaled along the upper side of the lower axis) increases. Note that the fall in oxygen parallels the fall in pressure only up to 12,000–15,000 feet, where greater increase in breathing sustains oxygen while "washing out" carbon dioxide more rapidly than at lower altitude. By deliberately forcing hyperventilation, alveolar oxygen can be kept higher, but carbon dioxide lowered perhaps to dangerous levels, at any altitude. The standard altitude/pressure curve is usually drawn with equal intervals along each axis and is a curve of decreasing slope. Here since the scales are different the dashed line is straight.

accumulates, breathing would be increased in order to wash out the excess. In fact, accumulation of carbon dioxide is a more powerful respiratory stimulant to breathing than is mild lack of oxygen: when you hold your breath at sea level, it is accumulation of carbon dioxide rather than lack of oxygen which forces you to breathe again.

Both lack of oxygen and excess carbon dioxide stimulate breathing, while lowered carbon dioxide slows breathing. An excess of oxygen, interestingly, seems to have no effect on breathing. These and other stimuli are read by a collection of chemo-sensitive cells in the midbrain called the respiratory center, from which appropriate corrective signals issue. Like the thermostat in your house that turns on the furnace when the temperature falls and turns it off when the house is too hot, the respiratory center responds to carbon dioxide and (to a limited extent) oxygen levels in the blood, and to changes in acidity of blood. This is an exquisitely sensitive and versatile feedback loop, responsive to blood and to spinal fluid (which is influenced, though only slowly, by changes in the blood). Another collection of cells, the carotid bodies, is responsive to oxygen lack and may take control of breathing at altitude.

Chapter Five

MOVING BLOOD: CIRCULATION

BREATHING MOVES AIR in and out of the lungs, and well-defined physical laws describe the passage of oxygen from lungs to blood and of carbon dioxide from blood to lungs. To ensure that oxygen is smoothly, continuously, and adequately transported to the tissues where it is most needed, we must have uninterrupted circulation of blood laden with oxygen. The circulatory system is as wonderful and intricate as the many other parts of our body, perhaps more so, since it is so largely self-regulating and autonomous. We may consider it in three parts: the pumping heart, the conducting blood vessels, and the transporting hemoglobin. The capability for adjustment in this system is a large influence on our ability to tolerate lack of oxygen.

The heart is the most immediately and obviously indispensable organ in the body because death occurs in six or seven minutes once the heart stops. By contrast, we may live for days or weeks with little activity of the kidneys or liver, and for weeks or months with an inactive brain. The heart is a marvelous and ingenious four-chambered pump. Poets and lovers to the contrary notwithstanding, all it does is pump, hour after hour, year after year, responsive to many stimuli yet able to function indefinitely without any outside intervention, spurred by its own intrinsic pacemaker. Though it is normally controlled by a network of nerves from many stations that read signals from throughout the body, the heart can be entirely self-governing. If every single nervous connection is cut, a tiny nucleus of nerve cells between the two thin-walled auricles (antechambers to the muscular ventricles — the pumping chambers) initiates the electrical stimuli which drive the pump at a steady, unchanging rate quite adequate to maintain life. It will continue beating so long as its needs for oxygen, nourishment, heat, and moisture are met, but at the same rate, unheeding of what the body may require.

Fortunately, the heart is seldom if ever called on to rely on this fail-safe intrinsic rhythm. If it were, we might exist quite adequately but we could not respond to the demands of exertion, the sudden spurt of fear, the relaxation of dreamless sleep, or to many other daily demands. The variety and freedom of life depend on the responses of the heart as stimuli come in from all over the body increasing or decreasing its activity. These stimuli pass through a control center in the hypothalamus which receives and evaluates nervous and hormonal signals from all parts of the body, switching them to appropriate centers that in turn send messages to heart and blood vessels.

Specialized receptors "read" the level of oxygen in the blood and signal the heart and blood vessels to take appropriate action, just as other centers direct changes in breathing. When blood oxygen falls, the heart is directed to speed up, to pump faster, and to increase the output of each beat. As a result, blood moves more rapidly through the lungs and to the tissues, supplying by speed the volume of oxygen it may lack. This is an emergency response, lasting for hours or a few days, during which other responses are triggered, and then the output of the heart returns to, and actually falls below, normal. Lack of oxygen is probably perceived mainly by small clusters of cells in the neck, the carotid bodies, which are richly supplied with blood, and with direct nerve communication to the hypothalamus.

Inadequate volume of circulating blood will also trigger corrective action: we call this condition hypovolemic (low volume) shock. The principal monitor of blood pressure is in the carotid sinus, another collection of cells, very close to but quite distinct from the carotid bodies. If blood pressure falls, or if we lose blood from hemorrhage, or if dehydration depletes volume, the heart is called on to pump faster and harder — again as an emergency response until the precipitating circumstances are corrected in other ways. The receptors for pressure and volume concern us little in our study of altitude hypoxia, but we know that they will be stimulated in the unwary climber who becomes dehydrated as he climbs higher, perhaps complicating the differential diagnosis between altitude sickness and hypovolemia.

Even though hypoxia stimulates the heart to beat harder and faster for a few days, blood pressure is not consistently affected by altitude. To be honest, the data now available are contradictory, with some studies showing that blood pressure in altitude residents and new arrivals is higher than normal, and other studies showing little or no change. We can say with modest assurance that blood pressure is probably little affected at altitude.

One protective change does occur to ensure that vital organs receive their necessary supply of blood: during hypoxia from any cause, particularly at altitude, blood tends to be shunted away from nonessential areas (skin, intestines, perhaps some organs) to those that are essential (heart, brain, and respiratory muscles). This too is a temporary compensation similar to the "dive reflex" that enables diving mammals to shut off blood from most of their bodies during periods up to an hour underwater — a truly amazing capability that man does not have.

Obviously the pumping heart must have conduits to convey blood throughout the body and back again; these vessels are called arteries, arterioles, and capillaries when they carry blood away from the heart, and venous capillaries, venules, and veins as they return blood from tissues — and from the lungs to the heart. The larger vessels have muscular coats (more pronounced in arteries than in veins), while the small capillaries are thin-walled to facilitate diffusion of oxygen and carbon dioxide. All vessels have a network of nerves that can, if necessary, dictate dilatation or constriction — a truly remarkable fallback protective system.

Man has always been curious about what made his heart tick. Writings that have survived for thousands of years show the extent of that curiosity and the ingenuity of explanations long before the microscope was invented and even before dissection was permitted.

In the western world, one of the first to recognize the pumping function of the heart and the role of the blood vessels was the versatile philosopher Empedocles, who likened the circulation to the ebb and flow of the tide, a concept accepted by Aristotle soon afterward. Aristotle taught that there were two different bloods: a "spiritual" blood, purified by passage through the lungs, and a "venous" blood, not so purified. He believed that the two mixed only to a limited extent, and then only by passage through almost invisible pores or holes between the two chambers of the heart. These beliefs were adopted by Galen five centuries later, became the official doctrine of the church, and prevailed for a thousand years.

Not surprisingly, the great Leonardo turned his mechanical genius toward the human body, meticulously detailing the leverages of muscles and, perhaps for the first time, recognizing (in 1500) that the heart was only a pump whose function was to move blood — a liquid which behaves like other liquids.

Another early pioneer was the Spanish scholar Michael Servetus, who trained first as a lawyer, then became deeply engrossed in religion; not till 1537 — at what was for those times the ripe age of twenty-six — did he take up medicine. As was common for scholars then, Servetus was interested in all natural processes and in their relationship to the divinity. He fell into conflict with the church, however, became a fugitive, and ultimately, pursued by the Inquisition (as were Galileo and Helmont), was apprehended while at church in

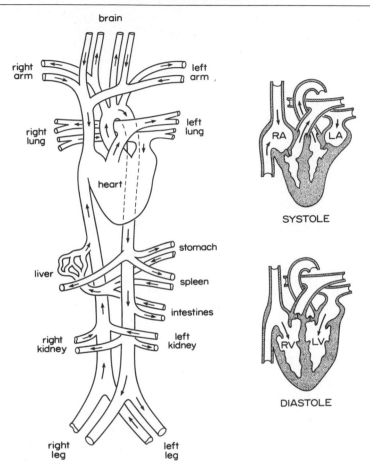

FIGURE 19. CIRCULATION: HOW BLOOD MOVES THROUGHOUT THE BODY

During systole (contraction), blood is forced out of the muscular left ventricle (LV) through the arched aorta into a system of arteries that feeds all parts of the body. At the same time, blood is pumped from the right ventricle (RV) through the smaller pulmonary artery into the lungs. During systole the smaller, thin-walled auricles (LA and RA) relax and are filled with venous blood returning (to the left auricle) saturated with oxygen from the lungs, and (to the right auricle) blood from all parts of the body containing carbon dioxide but depleted of oxygen. Then the ventricles in turn relax (diastole), valves between auricles and ventricles flop open, allowing blood to flow from each auricle into its adjacent ventricle. After the ventricles fill the cycle repeats. The left ventricle is a thick-walled, muscular chamber, capable of raising the blood pressure in aorta and arteries to 100–250 torr, while the less muscular right ventricle generates 15–40 torr in the pulmonary arteries. The auricles are weaker, generating only enough force to empty completely as the ventricles relax.

Galen understood most of this, though he believed that blood passed between the ventricles through minute pores in the wall between them, and that the lungs were a "dead end," as it were, serving only to cool the blood. Ibn al-Nafis, Colombo, Servetus, and many others added bits and pieces to this knowledge until Harvey was able to put them all together in his explanation of "The Motions of the Heart and Blood," which is how we understand the circulation today.

Geneva and speedily burned at the stake. Unorthodoxy, even in the name of science, was poorly accepted in those times. Servetus's great works (anonymously published in 1553, the year he was executed) were burned with him; three copies are known to have been saved, and from these it is clear that he understood very well the circulation of blood through the lungs, and dared to refute the great Galen (one of the "crimes" that led to his execution).

Two centuries earlier a Persian physician, Ibn al-Nafis, had also challenged Galen's pore theory. Though for religious reasons he performed no dissections, he theorized that blood leaving the right ventricle passed through the lungs and back to the left side of the heart and thence to the body, and that Galen's "pores" between the two ventricles did not exist, further postulating that the true purpose of the lungs was to aerate blood. He developed this theory five centuries before oxygen was discovered, but his manuscripts were lost until 1924, though there is some evidence to suggest that Servetus had heard of his ideas. Renaldo Colombo, who was developing the same theories as Servetus at about the same time, seems also to have known Ibn al-Nafis's work. Colombo's important book

De Re Anatomica was published in 1559, but as early as 1546 he was teaching a theory of blood circulation remarkably close to what we know today. Shortly after Colombo's book appeared, an Italian, Andrea Cesalpino, published a small treatise in which he stated that blood flowed from the right ventricle through the lungs to the left ventricle, and that valves in the vessels imposed unidirectional flow. Unfortunately, in his final book, published in 1606, he mistakenly described blood as flowing out from the heart not only in the arteries but through the veins as well. These speculations and observations laid the groundwork for the right man to assemble facts correctly and define how the heart and circulatory system function.

William Harvey was one of the parents of the scientific method and a pioneer in the young study of physiology. From Cambridge he went to Padua, then one of the great centers of medicine, where Vesalius first laid the foundations of the relationships between medicine, anatomy, and surgery. Galileo was also there and as Professor of Physics and of Mathematics undoubtedly influenced young Harvey's thoughts. Padua must have been an exciting place to study then, since it was well endowed and surprisingly free from bigotry, considering that the shadow of the Inquisition still lay across Europe. Harvey built freely on the work of Vesalius, postulating — though he could not see — the capillaries which permitted the flow of blood from arteries into veins in lung and all other tissues. He returned to London, entered private practice, and continued his dissections and lectures at the College of Physicians. Of his works by far the most important is *De Motu Cordis,* written in 1628 as a message to King Charles:

> *May I now be permitted to summarize my view about the circuit of the blood, and to make it generally known! Since calculations and visual demonstrations have confirmed all of my suppositions, to wit, that the blood is passed through the lungs and the heart by the pulsation of the ventricles, is forcibly ejected to all parts of the body, therein steals*

into the veins and the porosities of the flesh, flows back everywhere through those very veins from the circumference to the centre, from small veins into larger ones, and thence comes at last into the vena cava and to the auricle of the heart; all this, too, in such amount and with so large a flux and reflux . . . I am obliged to conclude that in animals the blood is driven round a circuit with an unceasing, circular sort of movement, that this is an activity or function of the heart which it carries out by virtue of its pulsation, and that in sum it constitutes the sole reason for that heart's pulsatile movement.

Harvey based his conclusions on the simple observation that both the valves within the heart and those in the veins would permit the blood to flow in only one direction. In his manuscript notes, which have survived since 1616, he calculated that the heart pumped in one hour blood weighing more than three times the weight of the whole body. His beautifully written *De Motu Cordis* may seem obvious today, but it was one of the great advances in anatomy and physiology.

How did Harvey synthesize so brilliantly when so many of his equally brilliant predecessors and contemporaries failed? One of his outstanding contemporaries, Robert Boyle, explained:

And I remember that when I asked our Famous Harvey in the only discourse I had with him (which was but a while before he dyed) What were the things that induced him to think of a circulation of the blood. He answered me that when he took notice of the Valves in the Veins of so many Parts of the Body, several were so Plac'd that they gave free passage of the Blood Towards the Heart, but opposed the passage of Venal Blood to the Contrary Way he was invited to imagine that so Provident a Cause as Nature had not Placed so many Valves without Design.

To illustrate the value of veins, Harvey used a picture identical to one which Fabricius had published twenty-five years earlier.

Four years after Harvey's death, Malpighi of Pisa, using the microscope, which had by then appeared on the scientific scene (whether first from Leeuwenhoek or Jannsen or Galileo is relatively unimportant), was able to see the capillaries, thus providing final proof of Harvey's theory.

The feverish growth of knowledge and the flowering of so many new ideas and the invention of such important new instruments, despite the heavy hand of dogma and the terror of the Inquisition, are never dull sources of wonder and inspiration. Though the exact composition of air and the essential role of oxygen had not been fully defined, the work of Borch, Mayow, Boyle, Hooke, and many others unsung today made possible the final contributions of Lavoisier and Priestley. Empedocles, Erasistratus, and Aristotle prepared the way for Galen, who was supplanted by Ibn al-Nafis and climactically by Harvey. After Jan Swammerdam and Leeuwenhoek described red blood cells, the way was open for Lower to establish that the major role of the lungs was to aerate blood and that something in air turned dark venous blood to bright red.

Chapter Six

TRANSPORTING OXYGEN: HEMOGLOBIN

THE PROCESSES OF breathing and of circulating blood about the body would be of little purpose unless there were a highly perfected means of carrying oxygen to every place it is needed and also for returning carbon dioxide from tissues to lungs for disposal. This part of the oxygen transport system is wonderfully accomplished by a simple but sophisticated carrier: the red blood cell, packed with hemoglobin. Our survival — especially at altitude — depends on the red cell just as much as it does on the breathing lungs and the beating heart.

Throughout recorded history, blood has been associated with life, even more so than air has been, perhaps because it is so highly visible and so easily spilled. In the fifth century B.C. the Greek philosopher-physiologist Empedocles wrote that "the blood is the life," and Aristotle believed that the soul depended on the composition of the blood. Their contemporary Anaxagoras was more specific: "The blood is formed by a multitude of droplets, united among them," a remarkable statement that seems to anticipate observations made by a Dutch lens maker two thousand years later.

Anton van Leeuwenhoek was not the first to use a magnifying glass: single lenses had been known for a century. But he was the first to combine lenses to make what we know as the compound microscope, which could magnify up to 300 times.

He was fascinated by everything small and estimated the size of the "little animals" (varieties of protozoa) as he did every other object by comparison with a grain of sand. He came astonishingly close to the 7.5 micra which we know today is the diameter of the normal, average red blood cell.

In 1674 Leeuwenhoek read a landmark paper to the Royal Society in London:

> *I have diverse times endeavored to see and to know what parts the blood consists of and at length I have observed, taking some blood out of my hand, that it consists of small round globules driven through a cristalline humidity of water; yet whether all bloods be such I doubte.*

These "globules" are not actually round but flattened discs, shaped like a doughnut whose center has not been punched out, and they are packed with a reddish stuff called hemoglobin — one of thousands of slightly different substances used by all living animals to carry oxygen from outside air to every cell. Different formulations of these colored compounds (called respiratory pigments) are used by different animals, depending on their particular needs. Most contain a few molecules of iron or copper bound to a pigment (porphyrin) and a species-specific protein (globin). Some animals use a simple solution of their unique form of pigment, but in most the stuff is contained in the small cells that Leeuwenhoek described.

There are thousands of different respiratory pigments with different affinities for oxygen. For example, most invertebrates use a substance that strongly attracts and holds oxygen, while in other species the attraction is rather weak. Tadpole hemoglobin attracts and holds oxygen very tightly, but as tadpoles become adult frogs this attraction weakens. The blood of animals living at high altitude — or in oxygen-poor environments, as do many marine animals — has a stronger affinity for oxygen than does man's blood. When the pigment is carried in solution (as it is in some animals), the "blood" tends to be thick and to move more sluggishly than when it is contained

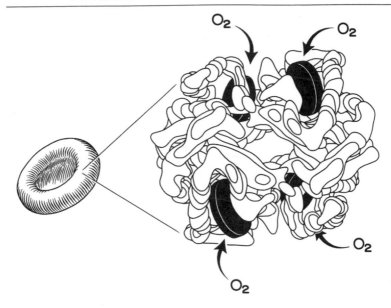

FIGURE 20. OXYGEN TRANSPORT:
RED BLOOD CELLS AND HEMOGLOBIN

The red blood cells, shaped like doughnuts with the hole not completely punched out, are packed with hemoglobin, a large and complex molecule containing four molecules of iron-containing heme, shown here in solid black. As oxygen enters the red cell by diffusion from the air sacs in the lungs, it combines with heme loosely enough for oxygen to be easily released as blood enters tissue capillary blood vessels surrounded by fluid and cells where oxygen pressure is low but carbon dioxide pressure high. Entry of carbon dioxide into the red cell helps to release oxygen. The contourlike lines in this illustration represent other components of hemoglobin that make it uniquely able to attract and release oxygen and to a lesser extent carbon dioxide under usual environmental conditions. Abnormal or mutant hemoglobins have slightly different arrangements of these molecules. Though they contain the same amount and form of heme, their association with oxygen and the shape they give to red cells are less favorable for man's normal life.

within cells. One can find persuasive evidence that such choices between solution and cells were dictated long ago by (or perhaps determined) the life-styles of all animals.

It is fascinating to find that the red substance containing iron, the particular combination we call hemoglobin, occurs widely throughout nature, though often in only a few species of one particular family, and in all of another related group. Almost all vertebrates have one of the thousands of possible hemoglobins, and so do some bacteria and even a few plants, though we can only speculate why. The hemoglobins are wonderfully built to combine loosely with oxygen when it is freely available (as where the partial pressure is high in the lungs or gills or whatever), and to release it easily to the cells where partial pressure of oxygen is low. We describe this almost miraculous characteristic by a curve relating partial pressure to the completeness with which hemoglobin is saturated with oxygen: the oxy-hemoglobin dissociation curve. It is perhaps one of the most important relationships in life, and we need to go back in history in order to understand it better.

Several years before Leeuwenhoek saw his little cells, Richard Lower had noticed that blood changed from dark red to a brighter carmine when agitated with air, but he did not know why. His contemporary Robert Hooke soon showed the Royal Society that an experimental animal could be kept alive when the chest was widely opened, so long as the lungs were rhythmically inflated. Lower, seizing on this, observed that blood changed from dark to bright red while passing through well-aerated lungs. Of course, oxygen had not yet been identified so no closer connection between breathing air and the change in blood was possible at that time.

In 1747 Menghini burned blood and showed that its ash was attracted by a magnet, which a century later led Justus von Liebig to speculate that blood contained some form of iron that carried oxygen, not in simple solution, but bound to an iron-containing compound within the red cells. Lothar Meyer soon showed this to be true, and in 1865 Felix Hoppe-Seyler crystallized this substance and showed it to his friend Paul Bert.

Bert was remarkably versatile: a lawyer, a plastic surgeon, and a politician. He studied under the great Claude Bernard, became interested in blood, oxygen, and high altitude, and wrote the seminal book on high-altitude physiology. In addition to his altitude studies, Paul Bert must also be remembered for his careful studies of how hemoglobin combines with oxygen. Using instruments he designed and had made, Bert exposed measured amounts of blood to different partial pressures of oxygen. He then used a vacuum pump to extract the oxygen which had combined with blood and was able to plot the relationship between oxygen pressure and the percentage of hemoglobin combined with it. From this he was able to draw the first oxy-hemoglobin dissociation curves.

Stated in the simplest terms, when blood is exposed to a high partial pressure of oxygen, most of it is immediately saturated, its iron molecules picking up molecules of oxygen. This happens in the lungs. When oxygen-rich blood reaches the tissues where oxygen pressure is low, the iron molecules quickly release oxygen, and the depleted blood returns to heart and lungs for another load. The shape of the dissociation curve dictates how fast and how completely oxygen is loaded and unloaded, and thus affects how animals tolerate oxygen lack.

Blood carries oxygen almost entirely in loose combination with hemoglobin; very little is in physical solution. Each gram of hemoglobin will bind or carry 1.34 milliliters of oxygen. Since there are or should be about 15 grams of hemoglobin in each 100 milliliters of blood, it follows that each 100 milliliters can carry 15 times 1.34 or about 20 milliliters of oxygen when hemoglobin is fully saturated. We call this the oxygen-carrying capacity of blood, normally described as 20 volumes percent. Changes in blood acidity, temperature, and carbon dioxide content change the carrying capacity.

When less oxygen is available, blood is less saturated. Though the *carrying capacity* is unchanged, the *actual content,*

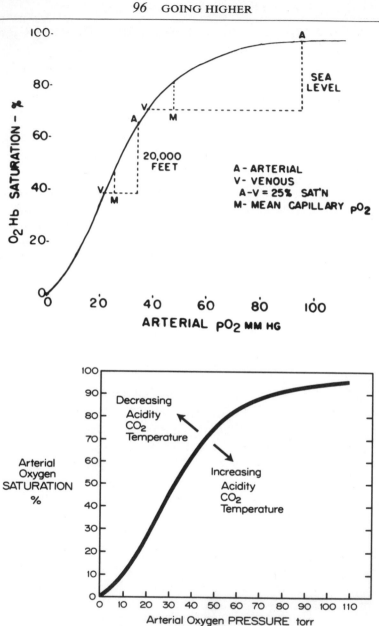

FIGURE 21. THE OXY-HEMOGLOBIN DISSOCIATION CURVE

Hemoglobin in red blood cells combines with oxygen in proportion to the partial pressure of oxygen in the surrounding air or liquid. When a curve is plotted relating oxygen pressure (abscissa) to percentage of hemoglobin which is saturated (ordinate), we find not a straight linear relationship, but a complex S-shaped curve. The characteristics of this curve are of the utmost importance (*upper left*): at higher levels of oxygen pressure (as at sea level), virtually all of the hemoglobin is saturated with oxygen, and even venous blood, returning to the heart after releasing adequate oxygen to tissues, is well saturated. By contrast, at high altitude (here shown as 20,000 feet), saturation falls considerably more for a smaller drop in oxygen pressure, indicating that a *volume* of oxygen nearly equal that at sea level can be released to tissues over a wide range of oxygen *pressures*. A similar curve constructed for hemoglobin removed from red cells does not have the S-shape and thus is a far less efficient oxygen delivery system. In the lower right-hand drawing, note how changes in acidity, carbon dioxide, and temperature change the inflection of the curve, thus altering oxygen acceptance or release.

---

or amount of oxygen carried, does change, being lower when oxygen pressure is lower. Capacity and content are the same only when enough oxygen is available to fully saturate the hemoglobin. Both capacity and content increase when hemoglobin is increased, and if hemoglobin increases in parallel to a decrease in available oxygen, we may have a normal oxygen content. So it is not surprising that an increase in circulating hemoglobin should be one of the ways in which man and some animals accommodate to lower oxygen in the air we breathe, and we will discuss this in the chapter dealing with acclimatization.

When Paul Bert drew the first rough curves describing the relationship between oxygen pressure and hemoglobin saturation, he could not measure some of the other influences that affect the curve. Nor could he fully appreciate the beauty of the special S-shape of the normal curve for human hemoglobin. We have made enormous strides since his innovative work and can better realize how admirably adapted to its task is hemoglobin.

In the lungs, where ample oxygen normally is available, hemoglobin becomes almost completely saturated. Even if the partial pressure of oxygen falls from 110 to 90 torr, blood is still 96 percent saturated, for we are on the flat part of the curve. This means that there is very little change in oxygen content up to about 5,000 to 6,000 feet. As oxygen pressure decreases (as we go higher), saturation begins to decrease: we reach the steeper part of the dissociation curve and oxygen is less firmly held. By the time blood has reached tissues — where oxygen partial pressure may be lower than 40–50 torr — it can hold less oxygen, and, most important, a small drop in pressure causes a larger drop in saturation, releasing a good deal of oxygen. The steeper the curve, the more oxygen will be released for a small drop in pressure. What a beautifully designed carrier it is!

The shape of the dissociation curve (and thus its ability to acquire and release oxygen) is affected by other things too, as Christian Bohr showed. Increasing temperature shifts the curve toward the right, while cooling moves it to the left. We can observe this in a crude way from how we react to very cold weather: the bright red cheeks and nose are probably due to the reluctance of blood coursing through the cold skin to surrender much oxygen, so it remains red. But the blue lips and nails of the shivering swimmer are due to the shunting of blood from skin to core in an attempt to conserve heat, and as a result the superficial blood is more depleted of oxygen even though this may happen more slowly.

Such shunting of blood from skin and less essential parts of the body to vital organs enables diving mammals to prioritize where oxygen is sent and enables them to stay so long underwater. Man may have a similar but weaker "dive reflex" responding to cold air — or water — by stimulating small nerve centers in the nostrils. But shunting is most useful for protecting us against excessive heat loss (hypothermia) and can have a harmful effect at high altitude where cold may cause shunting of blood already low in oxygen. This is a double insult to fingers and toes, and the danger of frostbite is thus increased by lack of oxygen at altitude.

Carbon dioxide also changes the shape of the dissociation curve. In the tissues, as carbon dioxide enters the blood, its increasing pressure shifts the curve to the right, but when it leaves blood in the lungs, its falling pressure shifts the curve back to the left. This Bohr effect increases delivery of oxygen to the tissues and assists oxygen acquisition in the lungs. Changes in acidity also change the shape: when blood is more acid the curve is flatter (right-shifted), and when more alkaline the curve moves toward the left. It is hard to imagine how a respiratory pigment could be better designed to serve man's wide-ranging activities and needs.

Hundreds of different or mutant hemoglobins occur in man, in perhaps half of one percent of all humans. The development of more sophisticated methods for analyzing the respiratory pigments has enabled identification of many subgroups of these abnormal hemoglobins, but most need not concern us here because they are laboratory curiosities, though a few are critically important.

One of these (S-hemoglobin) causes chronic anemia in about 0.3 percent of Americans; an additional 8–10 percent have what is called the "sickle trait" but are not anemic. The most common mutant form of S-hemoglobin has a slightly different molecular configuration than garden-variety hemoglobin; this exerts different stresses within the red cell and distorts some of the cells into sickle or half-moon shapes instead of the normal flat disc.

The sickle trait may become important at altitude because these stresses increase when S-hemoglobin contains less than normal oxygen, forming numbers of bizarre shapes which are less flexible and tend to stick like burrs in the narrow capillaries. Consequently, any cause of decreased oxygen, such as altitude, can cause problems due to obstruction of small blood vessels in the spleen and less often elsewhere, by these mis-shapen sickled red cells. Fortunately it is a rare problem, but one that can be serious if not recognized.

All of us have had three different forms of hemoglobin at different times in our lives. The embryo's blood contains a primitive form (P-hemoglobin), which soon changes to the F or fetal form, which has an affinity for oxygen much stronger than does adult or A-hemoglobin. This enables the unborn infant to pull oxygen more easily from its mother's blood passing through the placenta and thus helps the fetus to survive and grow in an oxygen environment comparable to that on top of Everest. It's really a useful extra means of acclimatizing to hypoxia. F-hemoglobin changes to the A or adult form soon after birth.

Some animals can switch back and forth between the F and A forms, for example, the high-altitude llama and the deer mouse, whose range is from sea level to 14,000 feet. Baboons have hemoglobin like man's, but they produce F-hemoglobin when they lose blood or are short of oxygen.

Much recent work suggests that we can modify hemoglobin to suit specific serious needs. One example (unfortunately too toxic to use except in an emergency) is a substance that stimulates formation of F-hemoglobin, replacing S-hemoglobin temporarily in sickle-cell crisis. Undoubtedly other, safer substances will soon appear, enhancing carriage of oxygen in persons where this is seriously impaired.

An ingenious substitute for red blood cells is already available: hemoglobin taken out of human red cells and packaged in plastic bags of the same size and with the same membrane characteristics as red cells. This "synthetic" blood keeps indefinitely, and since it contains only red blood cells in an innocuous solution, it causes none of the possible side effects that real blood may, but on the other hand it confers none of the benefits; it is solely an oxygen transporter.

The red cell is a selfless and versatile carrier: it has little need for the oxygen it carries and uses very little, which makes it a very efficient carrier. It has two other roles that are important at altitude: transportation of carbon dioxide from tissues to lungs, and regulation of the acidity of blood.

The acidity or alkalinity of blood (like any solution) depends on the amount of hydrogen ion (H+) or hydroxyl (OH−) in solution. The degree of acidity is indicated by the symbol pH, which is the negative logarithm of the concentration of hydrogen ions. A neutral solution (when both H+ and OH− ions are exactly in balance) has a pH of 7.0: the lower the pH, the more acid the solution and vice versa.

Our metabolism produces many acidic substances, such as carbon dioxide, lactic acid, fatty acids, and nucleic and uric acids. These could threaten the stability of the normal pH of 7.43 on which depends, as Claude Bernard said, our free and active life. When one realizes how many acids and how few alkaline substances enter the blood, the stability of the pH is all the more remarkable. It depends on several important buffers that can "absorb" H+ or OH− ions without much change in pH. There are six major buffer pairs in blood, three containing hemoglobin. But of these, the most immediately effective is the carbonate-bicarbonate pair, which is important in altitude physiology — and as a matter of fact in normal, everyday life because of the speed with which it can be altered by exhaling carbon dioxide or by excreting bicarbonate.

Carbon dioxide diffuses through capillary walls in the lungs and in the tissues some twenty times faster than does oxygen. Although only 10 percent is carried loosely attached to hemoglobin within red blood cells, this has an important effect on the transport of oxygen, as we saw above. Most of the carbon dioxide is carried in the liquid portion of blood (plasma) as bicarbonate, a substance produced by a reaction catalyzed by the enzyme called carbonic anhydrase. There is a high concentration of this in red cells, lungs, and kidneys — places where a shift in acidity can be speedily accomplished by changing the exhalation of carbon dioxide or loss of bicarbonate in the urine. The carbonate-bicarbonate pair is one of the more

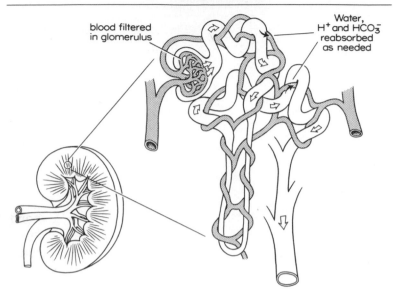

FIGURE 22. THE KIDNEYS

Arterial blood flows through capillaries around the glomeruli (filtration capsules) of each kidney. There are thousands of these and blood flow is large. By active selection the glomerulus allows water and many substances to pass through, entering a network of tubules which are surrounded by veins. Different parts of each tubule have different functions: in some sections water is absorbed; in others sodium, potassium, and other chemical compounds are taken in or allowed to pass under control of many enzymes, of which carbonic anhydrase is one. The selective filtration of the kidney is controlled by both nervous and chemical stimuli and in turn considerably affects the chemistry of blood, thus maintaining the constancy of the internal environment. Losing bicarbonate is one of the changes of acclimatization that improves tolerance for altitude. By inhibiting the formation of carbonic anhydrase, Diamox (acetazolamide) allows more bicarbonate to escape, thus (we believe) decreasing altitude illness.

mobile buffers in the blood. A substance called acetazolamide (Diamox) inhibits the action of carbonic anhydrase, and consequently has a strong effect on the acid–base balance of blood. This is discussed in chapter 9.

Of course, blood is far more than a simple vehicle for red blood cells: it contains other "formed elements" such as white blood cells and platelets that are essential to our well-being. A family of white cells called lymphocytes includes B cells, which make antibodies against infectious agents with the assistance of helper T cells, and killer T cells, which attack invaders such as tumor cells or viruses. Both B and T cells are affected by altitude, but curiously enough, different individuals respond very differently. Platelets are an integral part of the clotting mechanism and are increased during a long stay at altitude, though they may be decreased by acute exposure.

Blood also contains dozens of indispensable substances, some only in trace amounts, most in combination, and each has its own special function. Many have their own bioelectric potential or pump. Scores of hormones (messenger substances, unaffected by the messages they carry) have been identified, and there are doubtless many others. Blood transports foodstuffs such as proteins, fatty acids, and sugars, as well as the vitamins and enzymes which are necessary for their utilization. Blood carries waste products to be discarded by lungs, liver, or kidneys, as well as the immune bodies which protect against many invaders. Two other important functions which blood performs efficiently are regulation of temperature and maintenance of fluid balance. Although oxygen transport concerns us most in this book, the blood obviously has a great many other very important functions.

Blood is also an air conditioner: when we are too hot, the heat-regulating center diverts blood from core to skin where it may cool, and by increasing water loss in sweat may increase cooling further. Cold diverts blood away from skin to organs that must be kept warm if the body is to survive. Blood conserves water by shutting down urine formation and sweating when too much water has been lost; conversely, if we try to overload with water, blood facilitates its efficient discard in urine. Poems and novels and massive texts have described the wonders of blood; we can only deal with its function in oxygen and carbon dioxide transport.

Chapter Seven

USING OXYGEN: THE CELL

EARLIER IN THIS BOOK we looked at the intricate ways in which we acquire oxygen, transport it to the farthest parts of the body, and pick up and carry wastes to disposal sites. We peeked briefly at the complicated control network which maintains the constancy of our "internal environment" despite great fluctuation in the external temperature, pressure, humidity, and oxygen content. In our self-centered complacency we believe that this incredible mechanism has reached its pinnacle in man, even though a considerable part of our sophistication persists in trying to destroy all life.

All this network, all these activities are devoted to one end: the care and sustenance of individual cells. We breathe to acquire oxygen and remove carbon dioxide, and thus to ensure that every living cell has enough of one and not too much of the other. Our hearts pump in order that no cell lack oxygen and nourishment or suffocate in its own garbage. This "tiny bag of living water that floats in a great dead sea" (as William Bennett described the cell) is far more than a building block — it is life itself. Albert Claude, accepting a Nobel Prize in 1974, spoke lyrically about this tiny factory:

For over two billion years, through the apparent fancy of its endless differentiations and metamorphosis, the cell, in its basic physiological mechanisms, has remained one and the same. It is life itself, and our true and distant ancestor.

It is hardly more than a century since we first learned of the existence of the cell: this autonomous and all-contained unit of living matter that has acquired the knowledge and the power to reproduce; the capacity to store, transform, and utilize energy, and the capacity to accomplish physical works and to manufacture practically unlimited kinds of products. We know that the cell has possessed these attributes and biological devices and has continued to use them for billions of cell generations and years.

In addition, we know also that the cell has a memory of its past, certainly in the case of the egg cell, and foresight of the future, together with precise and detailed patterns for differentiations and growth, a knowledge which is materialized in the process of reproduction and the development of all beings from bacteria to plants, beasts, or men. It is this cell which plans and composes all organisms, and which transmits to them its defects and potentialities. Man, like other organisms, is so perfectly coordinated that he may easily forget, whether awake or asleep, that he is a colony of cells in action, and that it is the cells which achieve, through him, what he has the illusion of accomplishing himself. It is the cells which create and maintain in us, during the span of our lives, our will to live and survive, to search and experiment and to struggle.

*The cell, over the billions of years of its life, has covered the earth many times with its substances, found ways to control itself and its environment, and ensure its survival.**

With the powerful tools we have developed in the last few years we cannot only look at every tiny bit of the cell, but we can dissect out, alter, replace, or replicate the smallest fragments. One might think that no secrets remain hidden, but in fact most still evade us. With breathtaking speed our knowledge has accelerated, though our understanding lags behind. But think how far we have traveled since Robert Hooke first used the word *cell* before the Royal Society on April 13, 1663, when he used the newly developed microscope to demonstrate the compartments in cork. Though his microscope magnified

* Nobel Foundation. For permission to reprint I am grateful.

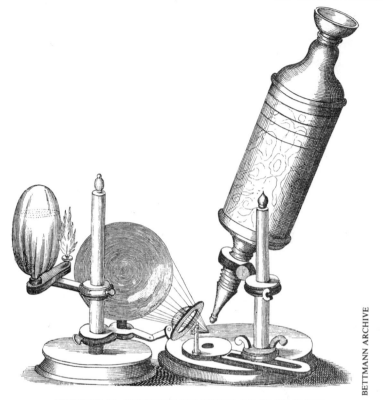

BETTMANN ARCHIVE

FIGURE 23. ROBERT HOOKE'S MICROSCOPE

Although Zacharias Janssen and Galileo developed microscopes between 1590 and 1610, the names of Anton van Leeuwenhoek and Robert
Hooke are more commonly associated with appreciation of the immense
value of that instrument. Leeuwenhoek made several hundred small
'scopes, some of which magnified over 250 times. Hooke's instrument
(*shown here*) was more complicated and gave finer detail and higher power.
With it he made thousands of drawings for his great book *Micrographia,*
which was one of the masterpieces of science in his century. Hooke was
charged by the Royal Society (then a fledgling club of the leaders of the
day) with preparing several new demonstrations each week, and his microscope helped him to fulfill this seemingly impossible task. The microscope
shown here magnified 400 times, and led him and others to studies
throughout the world of nature — both living and dead.

only 400 times, this was enough to show myriads of neatly arranged boxes, dead skeletons of houses once inhabited. About a century later, Henri Dutrochet, after looking at thousands of organisms, suggested that all living matter was made up of such individual cells, living cooperatively together, dying and being replaced. But living cells are made mostly of water and thus were difficult to study under the microscopes of those times, so Dutrochet's suggestion took some time to gain acceptance. Then Theodor Schwann, picking up some ideas advanced by Schleiden, demonstrated that the cell was indeed the basic structure of all living organisms, its life and death and organization contrasting sharply with the static structure of nonliving materials. We originate of course from the union of two single cells, each bearing elaborate instructions that direct the result of their union to grow into a human rather than a duck. But just how this is accomplished was explained only a few decades ago by the dramatic uncovering of the genetic code — the "double helix" made up of deoxyribonucleic acid, or DNA.

Even the best light microscopes of today depend upon light passing through or reflected from the object being studied and thus are limited in the detail they can reveal. About 1930 a sophisticated new tool was developed — the electron microscope — which in various ways makes it possible to distinguish individual molecules only a few angstroms in diameter. (The angstrom is 10^{-10} meters long, a very tiny measure indeed.) With this beautiful machine the most intimate structures can be examined, even the living cells of which we are made, and even while they function. Each cell is now recognized to be a complex community of more than forty tiny bits, each with a special function, each requiring nourishment and oxygen. Each cell is a minute factory where busy workers carry on their assigned tasks. Collections of cells form organs, different organs form the animal. Indeed, a living body is much like a city, where some sections are devoted to casting iron, others to baking bread, others to selling cars or beer, or making clothing.

The life of a great metropolis depends upon the interaction of these communities, each of which relies on thousands of individuals to make the food, provide power, or carry off the garbage, and each is a part of the humming whole. Just as a city can adjust to the loss of an industry, so the body can accept loss of, say, one kidney, or a part of its blood. Neither city nor man can lose many parts without dying. Neither the city nor the man can survive without a continuing supply of oxygen, and if their air is too depleted of oxygen, both city and human will die.

We have discussed how oxygen is brought to the smallest capillaries, where it flows "downhill" to its destination, the cell. Oxygen must pass through the red blood cell casing, traverse the liquid portion of blood, diffuse through the capillary wall and the fluid which bathes all cells, and finally it must enter the cell and reach the place where it is to be used: the mitochondria. Passage through the various membranes is dictated by physical laws: diffusion depends on the pressure difference or gradient across the membrane, the thickness, characteristics, and surface area of the membrane, and a coefficient characteristic of the gas or liquid and of the particular membrane, liquid, or space to be crossed. Though we can here consider only the passage of oxygen from blood to cell, the same principles apply to movement of any molecule through any medium, though of course the numbers are very different in each case.

But not all diffusion is so simple (if the above is simple!). Some cells are capable of "active transport," that is, they can use energy to move substances "uphill." Many substances are transported across membranes in our bodies, but the three we are concerned with (oxygen and carbon dioxide and water) are not. Though J. S. Haldane argued strongly that the alveolar membrane could actively secrete oxygen into blood, we have no evidence today that either oxygen or carbon dioxide crosses membranes by anything except passive diffusion, subject to the rules defined above.

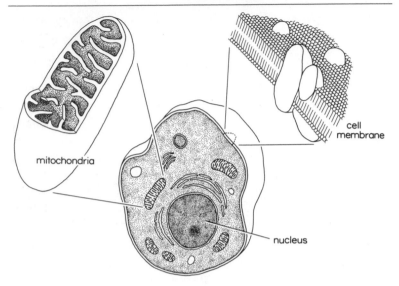

FIGURE 24. THE CELL: ITS MEMBRANE AND MITOCHONDRIA

The cell is the industrial park of the body. In it the mitochondria provide energy while other components recycle products, reproduce, or perform functions unique to each type of cell. A thin two-layered membrane encloses the cell, its molecules arranged in an orderly fashion like tadpoles with their tails facing inward and in constant motion, while between the two faces is an almost imperceptible space. Here and there in the membrane, larger molecules (also in motion) shoulder up as a substance moves in or out of the cell or remains a functioning part of its wall. The permeability or leakiness of the wall depends on a minute bioelectric charge which is affected by many things, including lack of oxygen. The cell membrane and the mitochondria (whose numbers vary from a few dozen to several hundred, depending on the type of cell) are most affected by hypoxia.

The integrity of life depends upon separation of "the bag of living water" from its surroundings by a membrane, and as Bennett describes this:

> *The boundary between a cell and the world is far more than a surface: it is a region that actively creates an interior different from all*

outdoors. . . . Cell membranes are not . . . featureless, efficient, smooth sheets — a kind of smart cellophane. They are studded with surface features which render the membrane as recognizable as a United States Marine in full dress uniform.

When we examine these surface features with our powerful instruments, we find that the cell membrane is a double layer of molecules, some oily, others water-soluble, stabilized here and there by cholesterol molecules and cobbled with large proteins, some associated with one face, others with the second face of the membrane, while still others penetrate both. These large protein molecules define the unique characteristics and functions of the different kinds of cells and provide "active transport" when that is called for. The membrane is about 100 angstroms thick, and its phospholipids, or fatlike molecules, are shaped something like tadpoles whose "heads" facing inward or outward present a compact surface, while their "tails" wiggle freely back and forth, keeping the layers in constant minute motion. The large protein molecules are also in motion, now and then shouldering their way up through the phospholipid heads, bulging outward from the cell here and inward there. The composition of these phospholipids is different in cells of different organs with different functions. Both layers of molecules carry minute electrical charges — the bioelectric potential. Currently the most plausible explanation of the impact of hypoxia on all or at least most functions is that lack of oxygen alters some bioelectric charges on cell membranes, thus interfering with transfer of sodium, potassium, and water into or out of cells. The aggregate impact of this disturbance may explain altitude illness.

Most simple gases, like other small molecules, pass through membranes as they do through space, by simple diffusion. Their molecules, darting here and there with incredible speed, rapidly scatter. No walls are completely impenetrable and the membranes of living tissue are selectively permeable, some allowing passage of only one type of molecule, others freely passing many different molecules.

Besides the pressure gradient and diffusion coefficient, another influence which greatly affects the speed and completeness of diffusion is the distance to be traversed. Cells may be immediately adjacent to capillaries, or separated by fluid or fibrous tissue, and the farther away a cell is from a capillary, the slower and less complete will be the movement of oxygen. Not many cells are far from capillaries, and one of the changes that contributes to acclimatization is the opening up of additional reserve capillaries, and even — after prolonged residence at high altitude — the formation of new ones so that very few cells indeed will be significantly distant from their oxygen supply.

There are thousands of different kinds of cells in the human body, each with unique capabilities and characteristics, each containing several dozen discrete parts. Two are of special importance in our search to understand how altitude affects the body: the genes and the mitochondria.

One of the most amazing accomplishments in medicine of the last quarter-century is our exploration of genes, the tiny building blocks arranged in neat designs to make up chromosomes that determine our unique individual characteristics. Chemically, genes are contained in long, double-stranded spirals of deoxyribonucleic acid (DNA), which control the formation of other substances in cells and thus dictate the genetic code. Only three simple substances (proline, serine, and glutamic acid), arranged in triplets, make up the "code words." Their placement or sequence in the double helix determines whether our hair is red or black, whether we tend to have depressions or are capable of genius, whether we may develop cancer or diabetes or live to be a hundred. If there is an inherited trait that acclimatizes generations to high altitude, it is carried by a special code word or words in the spiral.

In the last few years, incredible though it may seem, we have learned to rearrange the code words (at least in small organisms) and thus to change their characteristics and their functions. What such bioengineering may mean to the future bog-

gles the mind and has alarmed many. Genetic engineering may
be the most important capability man has ever acquired, for it
may perhaps be used to alter any living cell — in man, or bug,
or grain — and how wisely and well we use this power will
profoundly influence the future of life on earth if we do not destroy it first.

For our understanding of altitude illness and acclimatization, however, the most important bits in the cell are the mitochondria. In these intricate structures are made the molecules
of adenosine triphosphate — ATP — which is to life what electricity is to a motor: it makes it run. In response to an appropriate stimulus, the ATP molecule breaks down very rapidly,
releasing a very large amount of energy and forming adenosine
diphosphate (ADP). Three molecules of ADP are then slowly
reformed by a less energy-intensive process to make two molecules of ATP, and the process is ready to be repeated. Some
of these changes occur within and others outside the mitochondria. ATP breakdown to release energy is not oxygen-
dependent, but the rebuilding of ATP from ADP does require
oxygen and thus is likely to be affected by high altitude. Some
cells with many different functions have many mitochondria
(liver cells have 400), while others have few, like the single-
purpose sperm, which has only forty. Certain stimuli are believed to increase (or decrease) the number of mitochondria,
and one of these is oxygen lack. More mitochondria might
permit the cell to produce more energy by recycling more ATP
and ADP with less oxygen.

Mitochondria make the ultimate factory where fuel is
burned in the complicated cycles that energize every activity
including the creation of new cells. ATP is the molecular configuration in which energy is stored or released, used and re-
built, as ATP cycles to ADP and back. All life is dependent on
the ATP–ADP conversions, which we call metabolism. Even
though certain portions of it may take place in the absence of
oxygen, anaerobic reactions cannot be long sustained: oxygen
is necessary for completion.

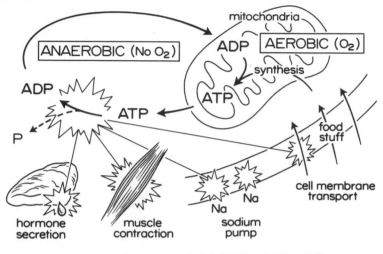

FIGURE 25. THE CELL'S METABOLISM AND
ENERGY PRODUCTION

After the food we eat has been processed in the stomach and intestines, the products of digestion (fatty acids, amino acids, simple sugars, and others) are passed through the intestinal walls into the blood and transported to tissues, where they enter cells either by simple diffusion or active energy-consuming transport. The liquid in the cell (cytoplasm) contains enzymes that further break down food substances for diffusion into the mitochondria, where energy production is centered.

There, under the influence of many enzymes arranged in an orderly fashion along the ridges of the mitochondria much like chemicals on laboratory shelves, these simpler substances are synthesized to adenotriphosphate, ATP, in a series of steps called the Krebs or citric-acid cycle. This process is oxygen-consuming, or aerobic. ATP is stored in the mitochondria and perhaps elsewhere, and whenever energy is needed it can be rapidly mobilized and instantly split, two molecules of ATP forming three of ADP (adenodiphosphate). This is a rapid, almost explosive release of energy that does not require oxygen (anaerobic). The energy released is used (1) to operate the sodium pump and to control passage of materials in and out of the cell; (2) to do work such as muscle contraction or secretion of hormones, among other tasks; (3) for the synthesis of various substances, especially the slower rebuilding of ATP from ADP, which depends upon oxygen.

These minute biochemical reactions, though immensely complex, are surprisingly well known. Lack of oxygen does not affect the quick release of energy in the anaerobic breakdown of ATP, but does markedly affect the rebuilding of ATP from ADP, which is oxygen-dependent. Perhaps this partly explains why sudden bursts of heavy work are possible at high altitude, while longer, sustained effort is not, and why recovery from work takes longer at altitude than at sea level.

After oxygen was identified and its role in combustion shown, scientists in the eighteenth and nineteenth centuries were greatly puzzled over how living organisms used food to create energy. How could mammals maintain the body at so constant and reasonable a temperature if food was being "burned" like a candle? (Equally intriguing was the question for cold-blooded or microscopic organisms.) Even the penetrating genius of Lavoisier and Priestley could not grasp how oxygen could be consumed and Joseph Black's "fixed air" or carbon dioxide be produced, without destroying tissue in which combustion occurred. Then in the middle of the nineteenth century Justus von Liebig showed how a metabolic process could produce controllable heat and energy without damaging tissues, and that in fact such control did exist not in the lungs, not in blood, but inside each living cell.

Louis Pasteur, responding to the pleas of French wine makers whose grapes were being ravaged by a mysterious malady (imagine the French losing their wines!), began to study fermentation and in 1858 showed that yeast was responsible. He believed that living yeast was essential, and not until 1897 when the Buchner brothers were able to ferment sugared water to alcohol with a cell-free extract from yeast was it clear that an enzyme, not the living cell, was necessary to make the cup that cheers. Thus began the studies which in the next seventy years deciphered the reactions by which foods are converted to energy. The Krebs or citric-acid cycle was defined, explaining how substances could be "burned" by the body without consuming it.

Intermediary metabolism has become a major discipline.

Microchemists have put together an elaborate diagram that pictures the Krebs cycle, yet it is still hard to visualize how such complex, intricate, and interdependent reactions can proceed most of the time with such efficiency. They have identified a number of diseases — mostly very rare — that are due to absence of a crucial enzyme. They have shown that certain poisons (notably synthetic pesticides) will block specific reactions or destroy essential enzymes. Other substances, such as acetazolamide, will temporarily inhibit other reactions. But for all the reactions that have been identified, hundreds, probably thousands remain to be understood completely.

The activities of every living cell in our bodies depend on oxygen. We have seen how the oxygen transport system ensures an uninterrupted supply — with small reservoirs in myoglobin and in blood to tide the cell over for a few moments. We can understand how the system and its reserves allow us to manage most activities. But man is capable of brief spurts of extreme effort, demanding more oxygen than can possibly be supplied quickly enough. We are able to exceed these oxygen-defined limits by emergency "switching" from the Krebs oxygen-consuming cycle to an anaerobic ("without oxygen") cycle. It is convenient (though not completely accurate) to think of this as a shortcut that can be used only briefly. Only for two or three minutes are we capable of "anaerobic work"; during this period we run up an "oxygen debt" which must be repaid, and no further work can be be done until the debt is repaid. During anaerobic work we can burn only glycogen (a complex sugar stored in muscles and the liver). If the supply has been drawn down by prolonged work or by fasting, we are less able to do anaerobic work, or even high-level sustained work.

Current wisdom for competitive athletes is to overload muscles and liver with a high-carbohydrate diet for a few days before competition, providing a better reserve to be drawn on after one and a half or two hours of demanding effort, and this is also true of climbers at altitude. However, whether this enables them to work along both the aerobic and anaerobic pathways at the same time is unknown.

Different organisms deal differently with prolonged hypoxia. We have seen how diving mammals conserve oxygen by shunting blood away from all but the most essential parts of the body, but we can still only speculate about their use of anaerobic pathways as well. Turtles may live for six months without renewing their oxygen supply, but when they surface and breathe air again it takes many days or weeks to repay the oxygen debt because they have lived with such a prolonged anaerobic cycle.

Substances pass the cell membrane (or any living membrane) in three ways. Simple diffusion depends on the difference in concentration on each side of the membrane, its area, thickness, and physical characteristics, and a few less important influences. Oxygen and carbon dioxide enter or leave cells by simple diffusion, dissolving in the fatty portion of the cell membrane. Water and many electrolytes probably go through tiny pores in the membrane. Water passes so quickly and easily in both directions that 100 times the volume of a cell moves in and out every second, yet normally the balances are so delicately regulated that the cell volume does not change. Electrolytes such as sodium, potassium, calcium, magnesium, and others equally important but in smaller traces are actively transported. Each has its own bioelectric pump, so that they move from an area of low concentration, uphill as it were, to an area of higher concentration. Glycogen and many other large molecules cross membranes by "facilitated diffusion," which means that they require a carrier and cannot enter the cell without one. I do not know whether or not hypoxia affects facilitated diffusion, but it seems likely that it does.

Of the many bioelectric pumps hypothesized (for of course they cannot be seen), that which moves sodium and potassium is thought to be most affected by hypoxia, for it is the most oxygen-demanding. The most persuasive explanation for altitude illness today is that the sodium pump falters and soon

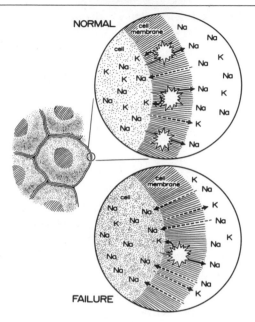

FIGURE 26. THE SODIUM PUMP

Each of our cells is enclosed within a delicate membrane through which can pass many substances, including sodium (Na), potassium (K), and water. Sodium tends to enter cells in larger amounts than does potassium, which tends to leave. To explain how the necessary delicate balance is maintained, an energy-intensive sodium pump has been postulated; this is oxygen-dependent and believed to use up to 20 percent of the energy each cell generates.

The sodium pump constantly pushes sodium ions out of the cell, while hindering the exit of potassium ions and allowing water to pass freely. In this way the concentration of sodium ions is kept lower inside the cells than outside, while the reverse is true of potassium. So long as the pump is functioning normally, osmotic equilibrium is achieved by passage of water in the appropriate direction. But if the pump falters or fails, as it is believed to do in several conditions, including hypoxia, then sodium is not pushed out as fast as it enters, while potassium leaks out. As a result, sodium builds up in the cell while the potassium level falls. To maintain osmotic equilibrium, water enters and the cell swells. Though these changes are extremely small, disturbance of the sodium pump and the resultant swelling of cells, most likely some more than others, is believed to be the basic cause of altitude illness. If true, this might explain why some symptoms are worse in some persons or on some days or in some organ systems. More swelling in the brain may cause the headache, more in the face may cause edema of the eyes, while swelling in other specific locations might cause the staggering walk, the hallucinations, or the accumulation of fluid in the lungs.

---

fails when deprived of oxygen. Since the concentration of sodium inside is one-tenth the concentration in the fluid outside the cell, the sodium pump must constantly push sodium "uphill" from low to high concentration. If it fails, sodium ions accumulate inside the cell. Potassium ions, normally more numerous inside than outside the cell, are constantly being pushed into the cell by the potassium arm of the pump. The sodium-potassium pump uses about 20 percent of the oxygen used by the cell and so is vulnerable when the oxygen supply decreases. As the pump falters, sodium accumulates within the cell, increasing its osmotic pressure and attracting water, which causes the cell to swell. We believe that this failure is the basis for many or most of the signs and symptoms of altitude illness, but it may be that other pumps (of which there are many) malfunction and also contribute to the problem.

More than half of the energy generated by the ATP–ADP cycle, called by the jaw-breaking term of oxidative phosphorylization, goes to housekeeping chores such as maintaining appropriate levels of electrolytes, water, food, and fuel to keep the cell alive and well. But each cell has other important functions too. Each must replicate itself before it dies. Some exist to detoxify the blood as the liver does. Others, in the kidney, excrete, reabsorb, or filter specific substances in response to commands from hormone messengers, themselves made by other highly specialized cells. Some cells make up the web of nerves and brain cells that generate, store, and transmit nervous signals, others make muscles contract or relax or digestive organs function. Each kind of cell is specialized, each has the requisite number and type of mitochondria, and each is enclosed in a membrane or membranes of special selective permeability. The activities of each kind of cell are dictated by the individual genetic code carried within its nucleus, and since each depends on oxygen for life, hypoxia affects them all. There is really no "typical" cell, but a very large number of quite different ones. Although each may have a similar overall composition, their response to oxygen lack varies widely.

Failure or weakness of the sodium pump is not enough to explain all the problems encountered at altitude, however, nor does pump recovery explain fully the process of acclimatization. The complicated cycle through which fuel is converted to energy requires a large number of enzymes as facilitators. Most are oxygen-dependent, and their functions are deranged unless sufficient oxygen is constantly available. But just how these contribute to illness or wellness is beyond the scope of this book. Barbashova, a distinguished Soviet scientist, has suggested that one of the adaptive mechanisms at the cell level is an increase in ability to do work with less oxygen (anaerobically), an ability that most tissues normally have to a strictly limited degree, when the immediate demand for oxygen briefly outstrips supply. Barbashova postulated that this increase in capacity for anaerobic work may be held in reserve while other enzyme systems gradually adapt to hypoxia. She calls the immediate reactions to hypoxia (such as increased ventilation and increased cardiac output) the "struggle responses," which sustain the body during the period of slow cellular adaptation. She places great emphasis on the observation that increased resistance of cells to hypoxia is not a response specific to hypoxia, but rather a general response that can be initiated by other agents as well. As Barbashova sees it, tissue adaptation plays a considerable part in acclimatization and is based on changes in enzyme systems and an increase in the number of mitochondria, which create more effective ways of using what oxygen is available.

Even so superficial a look at our human body as this has been leaves us marveling beyond words at the structure and function of these tiny cells, how they relate to one another to make a functioning whole, and how sensitive and resourceful they are in maintaining the constancy of our internal environment even when the external varies widely. The special cells that enable us to think about them, others that allow us to manipulate them, and still others that permit us to describe to other similar assemblages of cells what we see, hear, and think about them are beyond our power to comprehend. Even with all we know today we are only groping blindly with clumsy instruments to understand wonders which will never, ever be fully understandable. Man is not alone, not unique, perhaps not even the most intricate: billions of other organisms live and function with a variety of capabilities beyond our human limits. As we stand among the mountains, admiring their beauty, challenged by their size, let us pause for a moment to think of how even more marvelous is the organism that stands there marveling.

Chapter Eight

ALTITUDE ILLNESS

WHAT HAPPENS WHEN the carefully crafted mechanism for acquiring, transporting, and using oxygen, described in the preceding chapters, breaks down? Like most mammals, we require an almost uninterrupted supply of oxygen in order to live, and if the supply falters we too falter. Some hibernating mammals have evolved strategies for living with very little oxygen for weeks or months by slowing all their vital functions almost to a halt. Puny man, deprived of oxygen for as little as six to eight minutes, begins to die — from the brain down. We must have air.

There's a vast difference between what happened to the passengers on the ill-fated flight of the balloon *Zenith* and the dozen or so persons who have reached the same altitude on Mt. Everest breathing only the air around them. There is a smaller but still important difference between the flatlander who flies to a Colorado ski area and the instructor who lives there. The one is likely to feel miserable for a day or two, while the other has adjusted and feels almost as he does at sea level. Several factors determine whether you stay well or fall ill at altitude: how long you take to get there, how high you go, and how long you stay. There's a great deal of individual variation: because people are different they react differently. In general, the faster

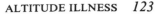

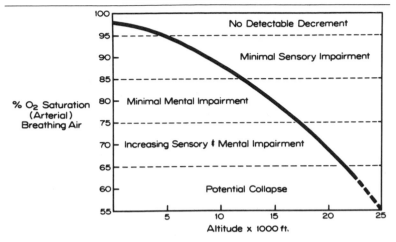

FIGURE 27. PHYSICAL AND MENTAL CHANGES
DURING RAPID ASCENT

If an unacclimatized person is taken up in a decompression chamber or aircraft at a climb rate of, say, 800–1,000 feet per hour, changes in some functions can be demonstrated as low as 5,000 feet — where dim-light vision is impaired. During the next 5,000–6,000 feet of climb, higher intellectual functions begin to falter: it becomes harder and harder to do simple arithmetic or puzzles or complicated tasks. By the time one arrives at 15,000 feet, handwriting is sloppy and thought processes become disordered and reponse to instructions slow or faulty. At 18,000 feet five out of a hundred healthy persons will collapse, and above 20,000 feet virtually everyone is appreciably and often comically altered, and more collapse. At 25,000 feet only a few moments of consciousness remain — if one has gotten so high! By contrast, consider the scores of Himalayan climbers who have lived and worked hard above this level, thanks to acclimatization (chapter 13). The percentage of oxygen saturation shown on the ordinate is only an average; it varies with over- or underbreathing and other influences.

you go and the higher you go, the more likely you are to experience symptoms.

Rapid ascent to great height is what killed Crocé-Spinelli and Sivel during the flight of the *Zenith* and almost killed many other rash balloonists of that era. In more recent times, interruption of their oxygen supply while flying too high has killed many unwary airmen. Sea level man taken rapidly to 18,000 feet is severely affected in ten to fifteen minutes, and five persons out of a hundred will be unconscious in less than half an hour. Taken to 25,000 feet he has only a minute or two of consciousness and less than an hour to live. A few unusual examples will illustrate how quickly lack of oxygen can kill:

One of the men working on the rim of a large vessel filled with nitrogen dropped a tool onto a platform three feet below the rim. He stepped into the vessel, stooped to retrieve the tool — and fell unconscious. His companion went in to get him out; he also died. There was only nitrogen in the vessel.

A teenager climbed down fifteen feet in an old well to rescue his dog, but before he could be pulled up he had died: at the bottom of the well carbon dioxide and marsh gas had displaced air, leaving little or no oxygen.

A scuba diver struggled to the surface after a shallow dive but was dead before rescuers could reach him: his dive tank was found to contain a lot of carbon monoxide, which bound to most of his hemoglobin, fatally interfering with oxygen transport.

This kind of acute episode doesn't happen on mountains, but it can happen to the high-flying balloonist or pilot who is totally dependent on his oxygen system: if this breaks down he may be incapacitated too swiftly to realize what has happened. At less extreme altitudes, if he fails to recognize loss of his oxygen supply, he will be impaired and may die, confused and thinking and performing irrationally. Lack of oxygen strikes the highest centers of the brain first — and thus judgment, perception, and recognition of one's danger are clouded early.

In some parts of the world the unwary visitor may have an unpleasant experience by going up so fast:

The telefero is a five minute taxi-ride from the airport (6,500 feet) and is in four sections. It takes about one hour to the top (16,500 feet). . . . Two of us went up from sea level . . . in about three hours. . . . I helped carry equipment . . . and was feeling quite well all afternoon. Then I felt worse and worse — bad headache, lack of energy and very tired. I seemed to feel better if I consciously tried to breathe deeply. . . . I had a couple of bowls of soup and a candy bar . . . slept for about 30 minutes, and woke and immediately lost the soup. Back to sleep and repeat the performance in half an hour. Morning came finally and I just didn't have any energy. . . . Still had my bad headache but as we descended in the tramway I felt better and better and by the time we reached the bottom . . . I took my suitcase and walked to the airport (a couple of miles).

We are concerned with more gradual exposure — slower ascent to less dangerous altitudes and less dramatic outcomes. The mountaineer, the skier, the trekker, and the casual tourist who go above 8,000 or 9,000 feet in a day, or the mountaineer who goes too fast to 14,000 feet, are the ones to whom this lesson is addressed.

Scientists like to classify in order to better understand what distinguishes birds from bats or frogs from toads, and a few conventions will be helpful as we look at altitude illnesses. For the last twenty years most people have divided altitude illness into four categories: Acute Mountain Sickness (AMS), High-Altitude Pulmonary Edema (HAPE), High-Altitude Cerebral Edema (HACE), and Chronic Mountain Sickness (CMS). Some prefer terms like Benign Mountain Sickness and Malignant Mountain Sickness, depending on the progress and severity of symptoms. Others believe all should be classified as Acute or Chronic Mountain Sickness.

Despite these reservations, we can make a useful classification of signs and symptoms that will help to identify the severity of illness, help to decide what treatment is best, and improve our studies of the epidemiology of this preventable problem. Here is the one most generally accepted.

- *Acute Mountain Sickness (AMS):* called *puna* or *soroche* in South America. Afflicts 15–17 percent of people who go too rapidly to 8,000 feet or higher. Characterized by headache, fatigue, shortness of breath, disturbed sleep, sometimes nausea and vomiting. Self-limited and rarely requires treatment or descent.
- *High-Altitude Pulmonary Edema (HAPE):* Occurs above 9,000 to 10,000 feet (rarely lower), usually taking thirty-six to seventy-two hours after arrival to become obvious. Shortness of breath and cough are severe, and frothy or bloody sputum is likely. Headache, great fatigue, sometimes slight fever develop. Sometimes mistaken for flu or pneumonia. May progress rapidly to coma and death. Probably most people develop very mild lung edema soon after arrival but the fluid is usually reabsorbed quickly.
- *High-Altitude Cerebral Edema (HACE):* May occur as low as 9,000 to 10,000 feet but usually higher. Usually develops insidiously over twenty-four to thirty-six hours. Ataxia is an early sign; mental confusion and hallucinations are common. Some degree of HACE may occur in all forms of altitude illness, but in pure form it is rare.
- *Chronic Mountain Sickness (CMS):* Often called Monge's disease. Affects a few persons resident at altitude who fail to acclimatize to or — more often — lose their tolerance for altitude. Fatigue, chest pain, ruddy (plethoric) appearance, and greatly increased red blood cell count and heart failure result. Though relieved by blood-letting or descent to sea level, death results if the patient remains at altitude.

Some include all altitude illness except CMS under the umbrella name of Acute Mountain Sickness, treating HAPE and HACE as complications. They argue that all are due to oxygen lack and that one often leads to another. To me this is confusing and I prefer the above classification. Regardless of terminology, we know that lack of oxygen is the root cause, and that the manifestations are not separate diseases but parts of a continuous spectrum in which now one, now another may dominate. We believe hypoxia causes reversible failure of the sodium pump, which makes cells unable to handle water and electrolytes normally. This is described in chapter 7.

But there is more, much more, to altitude illness than this. Disturbed blood flow to the brain, due probably to changes in blood acidity caused by overbreathing, certainly contributes to symptoms of AMS. Brain tissue is so tightly packed into the rigid skull that even a small change in its volume (whether due to greater blood flow, or to swelling of its cells) will cause signs and symptoms, discussed in chapter 11. The lungs are so built that changes in blood pressure and flow initiate release of a number of biologically active substances which contribute to pulmonary edema, as is discussed in chapter 10. Changes in enzyme activity and in the messenger hormones contribute to the process of acclimatization, and if these are inadequate, then altitude illnesses of one type or another result. Let us look in more detail at some of these hormones and enzymes, for they are made in the body and are essential to everything we are and do.

If you ask people to associate the word *hormone* with some other word or function, many will respond with *sex* because hormones are probably best known for the roles they play in sexuality and reproduction. If you ask what an enzyme is, most people think of yeast and fermentation or digestion. But scientists tend to be a little vague about precise definitions because our expanding knowledge has blurred the differences between the two.

Originally *hormone* meant messenger, derived from the Greek verb meaning to stimulate, to excite, or to set in motion. The god Hermes was the Greeks' messenger, in charge of commerce and invention — and also of thievery and cunning. Our hormones are in fact messenger substances, usually manufactured by one group of cells (endocrine glands) and carried by blood or other body fluid to their target organs, which they stimulate into action. The best known are those made by the pituitary, the adrenals, ovaries, testes, the pancreas, and the thyroid and parathyroid glands. Recently an important group of cells that secrete a hormone which has a powerful effect on the flow of urine has been found in the heart muscle; presumably these cells respond to changes in pressure or volume of the heart. Every hormone has its own very specific task and controls specific functions.

Scores of hormones are known and many of them have been synthesized. Many must be triggered by a "release" hormone and their secretion halted by an "inhibitor." Many, perhaps most, are secreted in regular rhythms. The female hormonal cycle, for example, is approximately four weeks, and some believe that male hormones have a less evident cycle of different length. Secretion of adrenal and pituitary hormones is known to fluctuate regularly during a day, each peaking at a different hour so that their action waxes and wanes. Circadian rhythms (as the cycles are called) are not fully understood despite a great deal of research, but we do know that resistance to disease or effectiveness of a medicine is greater at some periods of the day or night than at others. It is likely that similar fluctuations occur in man's resistance to hypoxia; this has been demonstrated in animals. This relatively unknown area is more important than we recognize today.

Less well known are the substances which are made and act locally, such as those which make possible the passage of a nervous impulse from one nerve ending to another, or which control impulse transmission within the brain. These are called neurotransmitters, but they are more like enzymes than hormones.

Enzymes are far more numerous and more complicated. More than a thousand have been identified and undoubtedly tens of thousands more exist in anonymity. The word *enzyme* also comes from the Greek, from a word meaning "fermentation"; Pasteur chose the word deliberately to describe the active principle in yeast which makes wine or beer from fruit or grain. Enzymes are catalysts, accelerating, often greatly, chemical reactions in which they are themselves not changed. Deficiency of a specific enzyme will cause a specific defect such as phenylketonuria (PKU), much as lack of a hormone causes identifiable illness like hypothyroidism or diabetes, and as aging alters the female hormones which control menstruation and fertility.

Twenty or thirty years ago the distinction between hormones and enzymes seemed clearer than it does today because so many substances have recently been identified which seem to fall between the two. Some are produced in response to a local stimulus and survive for only a short period of intense activity before being converted into other active substances. Among these are prostaglandins, identified fifty years ago but only recently appreciated by the award of three Nobel Prizes for their discoverers. Prostaglandins are present in almost every part of the body and have a vast range of activity. Leukotrienes, thromboxanes, and dozens of substances active in accelerating or preventing blood clotting are others in this category. A great number of enzymes take vital but often fleeting roles in the chain reactions called the Krebs or citric-acid cycle, by which cells use fuel to create energy.

There is a tendency today to think of enzymes and hormones and these others as "biologically active substances," leaving precise definitions to taxonomists, because the distinctions are sometimes blurred.

At least a nodding acquaintance with hormones and enzymes is necessary if we are to discuss altitude adequately, because they are undoubtedly more influential in determining illness or wellness at altitude than we recognize today. Unfortunately, many of these biologically active substances are elusive and their action fleeting, and they are affected by so many external influences that controlled studies are extremely difficult. The published literature contains many contradictory reports and is, to say the least, difficult to understand.

Fortunately, a few things are clear. At altitude (and, by extension, during hypoxia from other causes as well), these changes occur:

- Renin (made in the kidney) is released and activates a series of substances called angiotensins, which stimulate release of aldosterone from the adrenal glands.
- Angiotensin II is a powerful vasoconstrictor and probably increases pulmonary artery blood pressure, although it usually has less effect on blood pressure in the rest of the body.
- Antidiuretic hormone (ADH) is secreted by the pituitary and in some circumstances causes fluid retention.

All these events are damped by time, by inhibiting hormones, by the induction (meaning stimulation or formation) of enzymes which break down the hormones, and probably by the time of day, diet, exertion, stress, and many other influences. Hormones and enzymes also act upon each other. This is what makes controlled studies so difficult.

Within the lung (and almost surely elsewhere as well) other substances are released or formed (prostaglandins, thromboxanes, leukotrienes, etc.) which have powerful effects on blood vessels. Some neutralize others, and the balance between opposing actions seems to determine whether or not one succumbs to an altitude illness like HAPE, for example.

James Milledge, Michael Ward, and Edward Williams have shown that strenuous exertion at sea level mirrors many of the hormonal interactions that are triggered by lack of oxygen at altitude. Milledge suggests that the renin-angiotensin-aldosterone system is set in motion by exertion just as it is by hypoxia, causing sodium and water to be retained in the cells and potassium to be lost, thus causing edema. Those persons who only slowly or weakly develop mechanisms inhibiting these hormonal changes are vulnerable to altitude illness just as they are to exercise edema, while those with stronger defenses are not. Acclimatization includes, among many adjustments, strong inhibition or neutralization of the sodium- and water-retaining hormones, as well as enhancement of the enzyme systems within the cells. This is discussed further in chapter 13.

There is a huge difference in susceptibility from one individual to another, and a person may be ill on one occasion and yet perfectly well on another, apparently in similar circumstances. We have learned that many people have problems that take care of themselves, while in others a seemingly mild case of AMS may develop into HAPE or HACE and become life-threatening:

Because of headache, cough, and difficulty sleeping, a thirty-one-year-old man consulted a doctor forty-eight hours after arriving at 9,500 feet; he was thought to have "flu" and told to go to bed and take aspirin. Next day he returned with considerable shortness of breath, cough, and signs of congestion in his lungs. He was irrational and disoriented. He was found to have pulmonary edema and early cerebral edema and was sent by ambulance to a lower altitude, where he recovered rapidly.

Some who ignore the warning signs are not so lucky:

A healthy airline pilot reached 9,500 feet several days after leaving sea level. Despite increasing nausea, weakness, shortness of breath, and confusion, he continued to ski. On the third day he was unable to put on his skis, staggered and fell when walking, and left his wife and friends to go to bed. Next morning he could not stand, rapidly became comatose, and had a cardiac arrest as he arrived at a medical clinic. He was resuscitated and flown to an intensive-care hospital, but he never regained consciousness and died twelve days later.

Although he had told his wife he would visit a doctor when he left the ski area, he did not do so. This tragic death could have been avoided if he or his companions had recognized the clear warning signs of severe altitude illness. It's interesting that no one else in the party had symptoms, although they had come up together and had done the same things.

Inability to handle salt and water is a result of hypoxia, and sometimes this may be inadvertently exaggerated.

A young woman felt miserable during the first two weeks of a visit to a resort at 8,000 feet. She gained almost twenty pounds and her entire body felt swollen. Inquiry revealed that her physician had advised her to eat plenty of salt. She had done so and had also taken more water, and because of the altitude had not been able to handle the increased load. Drastically reducing her salt intake caused a prompt loss of this "water weight" and disappearance of symptoms.

Hackett and his colleagues found that 18 percent of trekkers passing through the Himalayan Rescue Foundation clinic at 14,000 feet had swelling of the face, hands, and feet and were retaining abnormal amounts of water. This group also had more symptoms of altitude illness than did those without edema. Quite possibly the heavily salted Tibetan tea, served at all the teahouses along the route, may have contributed.

Although we are confident that lack of oxygen, and the resulting difficulty handling water and salt, is the basic cause of altitude illnesses, it is hard to understand why some persons in a party are unaffected while others are very ill, or why one person may be ill on one occasion and not on another, apparently similar, climb. Nor do we understand why signs and symptoms seldom appear for several hours or even longer after reaching moderate altitude. This puzzled Ravenhill, a physician to a mining company at 13,000 feet who in 1913 wrote one of the finest descriptions of altitude illness:

It is a curious fact that the symptoms of puna *do not usually evince themselves at once. The majority of newcomers have expressed themselves as being quite well on first arrival. As a rule, towards the evening the patient begins to feel rather slack and disinclined for exertion.*

Why should this be? Angelo Mosso hypothesized that the increased breathing — which is a natural response — not only increased oxygen in the lungs but also decreased or washed out the carbon dioxide, and that rather gradual loss of carbon dioxide (for which he coined the term *acapnia*) might cause many of the symptoms attributed to oxygen lack. A neat idea perhaps, but some of those worst hit by HAPE or HACE actually breathe less than normally and their blood carbon dioxide levels are higher rather than lower than at sea level.

Another hard-to-explain observation based on a great deal of experience in the mountains is that taking a victim down even a few thousand feet seems to do more good than giving him oxygen. This is quite unexpected, and if the observation can be confirmed by carefully controlled studies, it would suggest that Mosso's idea might have some validity, or that decreased barometric pressure, quite independently of lowered oxygen pressure, is somehow involved.

We know that the level of oxygen in the blood is not always directly related to the presence or absence of symptoms. So we are forced to conclude that other factors than we now recognize are working on us at altitude; we simply do not have all the answers. This does not change our certainty that going too high too fast is likely to cause problems for many people, and that lack of oxygen is the primary cause of all forms of altitude sickness.

Although we consider the various forms of altitude illness parts of a continuous spectrum, each does have unique features, which we will look at in the next few chapters.

Chapter Nine

ACUTE MOUNTAIN SICKNESS (AMS)

SEVERAL YEARS AGO the Snake River Health Service (a non-profit medical clinic) conducted a survey of visitors to six Colorado ski areas, all at 8,000 feet or higher. Three thousand nine hundred and six persons were interviewed, most of them having arrived from low altitude within a day or two. Of those, 17 percent were having symptoms at the time, which they attributed to altitude, and 12 percent had three or more of the symptoms thought necessary for a diagnosis of AMS. Fourteen percent said they had had altitude sickness before, at, or below 9,300 feet. Only people who were up and around were questioned — which means that those who might have been sicker were not included. No effort was made to exclude those who might have some other problem, like a hangover or a bad cold, but despite these epidemiologic weaknesses, the study probably represents a good estimate of the percentage of visitors likely to be afflicted.

These findings are similar to those of other studies, in the Himalayas and the Andes, where the incidence of illness was higher at higher altitudes. The Colorado figures have some interesting economic consequences:

Anyone who has had even mild AMS knows that it causes one to lose interest in food and drink and even in sex: the temptation is to mope around feeling sorry for oneself and waiting to get better or die.

From this we could reasonably assume that AMS might keep a person from spending a bit of money on food or drink or skiing. Now we don't know exactly how many tourists from the flatlands visit these resorts, but a good guess is that more than half of the 25–30 million tourists who visit Colorado annually go up into the mountains. If 12–15% of these each refrain from spending $25 because of feeling miserable, we are looking at a loss to resort owners of 50 to 60 million dollars a year. This does not include those who are really sick, those who go home early, or vow never to come again. Clearly this is more than a minor medical nuisance — it's a major economic matter.

Because millions of people go to moderate altitudes like 8,000 to 10,000 feet all over the world, we are talking about a common illness with large human and financial impact. Two vivid descriptions come from the last century, though the victims were taken ill above 10,000 feet. Edward Whymper, conqueror of the Matterhorn and the most famous climber of his generation, wrote in 1876:

I found myself lying flat on my back . . . incapable of making even the least exertion. We knew the enemy was upon us and that we were experiencing our first attack of mountain sickness. We were feverish, had intense headaches and were unable to satisfy our desire for air except by breathing with open mouths. Headache for all three of us was intense and rendered us almost frantic or crazy.

Whymper tended toward drama, but he and his party had climbed quite high and were hard hit by AMS. Edward Fitzgerald, his famous contemporary, was equally affected during the first ascent of Aconcagua in the Andes, even though the party had taken many weeks for the climb, and in 1899 described it thus:

I was only able to advance one or two steps at a time, and then I had to stop, panting for breath, my struggles alternating with violent fits of nausea. At times I would fall down, and each time had greater difficulty rising; black specks swam across my sight; I was like one walking in a dream, so dizzy and sick that the whole mountain seemed whirling about me. . . . As I got lower my strength revived, and the

*nausea I had been suffering from so acutely disappeared leaving me
with a splitting headache . . . so bad it was with great difficulty I could
see at all.*

J. S. Haldane, the most distinguished physiologist of his
time, made some more restrained but telling observations during the Pikes Peak expedition of 1911:

*Among numerous visitors who came up by train and stayed only
about three quarters of an hour . . . there was as a rule no marked discomfort but some persons became very miserable and faint, and actual
fainting was observed occasionally as well as vomiting. Among those
who walked up or came up on donkeys the symptoms were much more
general and severe. The blueness was more marked and nausea and
vomiting, headache and fainting were extremely common. . . . The
scene in the restaurant and on the platform outside can only be likened
to that on the deck or in the cabin of a cross-channel steamer in rough
weather.*

Butchers, bakers, candlestick makers, men, women, and
children, young and old can and do get just as sick as distinguished climbers and doctors. AMS usually begins with headache that grows worse and worse, pounding "like a devil's
anvil," aggravated by straining, coughing, or lifting, and little
improved by aspirin or similar remedies. Some describe it as a
tight band compressing the skull; others feel their head is about
to burst. It is as bad lying down as standing but is slightly improved by mild exercise. It is the most common and unpleasant
symptom, lasting for several days before gradually going away
unless the victim persists in going higher.

Insomnia is another frequent symptom, compounded of
course by headache. Even without headache, restless or absent
sleep is common for many nights after arrival. Irregular or periodic breathing, often called Cheyne-Stokes breathing, is
common above 9,000 feet and certainly makes sleep more elusive. Just as the victim is dozing off, a snort or a snore signals
the end of a period of little or no breathing (apnea). Then

comes a series of increasingly deep gasps, a decrease, and again apnea. This is very disturbing to one already restless!

Weakness, lethargy, easy fatigue are typical. The energy level is low; it becomes an effort to do anything, even though light exercise often makes the sufferer feel better. Shortness of breath (dyspnea), though usually not very severe, is enough to dampen thoughts of exertion. If dyspnea or headache is especially bad, it is likely to indicate something more serious.

Loss of appetite (anorexia) is also common. Even favorite foods lose their appeal, and some unusual items may be craved — but soon are unwanted. Anorexia goes hand in hand with lethargy; loss of weight results. Sometimes nausea and vomiting complicate matters.

Sometimes there is so much swelling of face, hands, and feet that a person is unrecognizable or may be unable to put on boots. This inability to handle water normally is typical, but it can also occur at sea level during and after strenuous exertion.

For a week Dr. Michael Ward and friends walked for six or eight hours a day in North Wales, never getting higher than 3,500 feet. They carefully measured their food and water intake and urine output and made a number of blood measurements as well. Of course they didn't have AMS or HAPE or HACE, but they did develop water retention, and a good deal of edema, especially around the eyes and in the ankles. Perhaps inability to handle salt and water normally at altitude is due at least partly to what Ward called "exercise oedema," the result of abnormal secretion of hormones.

AMS is much like a bad hangover and like a hangover usually subsides in a day or two, though it may persist or even develop into full-blown HAPE or HACE. It is unpleasant, sometimes prostrating, and common among visitors at 8,000 feet. Headache is a frequent complaint among mountaineers arriving at base camp on Everest or K-2, or at the Mt. Logan High Altitude Laboratory — all of which are over 17,000 feet — even though climbers have taken many days or weeks for their ascent. Periodic breathing strikes almost everyone above 10,000 feet, and "white nights" when one scarcely sleeps at all are usual above 19,000 feet. Lethargy adds to the problems of getting up on a bitterly cold morning in a cramped and frozen tent. Loss of appetite and craving for bizarre foods is a big challenge for those planning meals on high mountain expeditions. But should we call these AMS? I think not.

It is not surprising that altitude affects mountaineers on very high peaks, but the visitor to a mountain resort is also a frequent victim: what can we learn from him? Perhaps there is a message that we are failing to read in the fact that symptoms do not begin immediately on arrival and actually may not develop for several hours, as Ravenhill recognized back in 1913. Yandell Henderson made similar comments during the expedition to Pikes Peak a few years later:

For the first hour or so after arrival we were all very cheerful, unpacking apparatus and fitting up the room that was to be our laboratory. Then one after another my three comrades began to exhibit in their mental attitude the blueness which was already a striking feature of their lips and faces. Dinner did not interest them; society was not wished for. The question which seemed principally to concern them was whether they should take themselves to bed or in the language of the ocean liner should "go to the rail."

As is the case with so many other illnesses, understanding the causes of a problem is the first and biggest step toward prevention. On Mt. Kenya, Mt. Rainier, and in the Himalayas, even though more people seem to be climbing, the incidence of all forms of altitude illness has decreased as people become knowledgeable about the risks and take appropriate precautions.

They have learned (or are beginning to learn) that the best prevention is to go up slowly. Taking a day to ascend each 1,000 feet above 5,000 or 6,000 feet will protect most people. Because breathing is shallower and less regular during sleep, we get less oxygen then, especially at higher altitudes. So the mountaineer has learned to "pack high and sleep low" — good practice for anyone going above 12,000 feet, and helpful lower down. This partly explains why more people aren't ill on ski hills: although they may ride the lift over and over again to 12,000 feet during the day, they generally sleep much lower.

On major mountain expeditions the climbers may take many weeks for the approach march, climbing up and down many ridges before reaching base camp, usually higher than 17,000 feet. Such large expeditions laid siege to a mountain, carrying huge amounts of equipment to base camp and laboriously ferrying this up to successively higher camps. As each camp was stocked, the climbers moved to the next, leap-frogging toward the summit. They were able to ride out storms, and a secure escape route was left below them; their acclimatization improved — but only to a point, because above 20,000 feet they lost weight and strength, and even the will to go on was eroded. These huge expeditions often reached a summit, but they were beyond the reach of many young climbers.

So the small party, relying on strength and speed and skill rather than weight and numbers, was a logical next step. Many of these parties are ultra-light: three or four climbers trek to 16,000–18,000 feet and make acclimatization climbs in the vicinity. When conditions are auspicious they start their chosen route, perhaps fixing ropes to move up swiftly later on, perhaps leaving supplies at several sites. Acclimatizing rather than deteriorating at base camp, they will wait for settled weather and then make the dash for the summit. These talented men and women often climb 8,000 or 10,000 feet or more in two or three days, often over difficult and dangerous routes, carrying little. The risks of exhaustion, frostbite, dehydration are large, but even more subtle and dangerous are HAPE and HACE. The challenge is to get up and down before these became incapacitating or life-threatening. And often these intrepids win! But there are many losers, brilliant, experienced, talented people who die of pulmonary or cerebral altitude illness, often during descent.

Taking time is best, but even so, some people will have problems. We don't know why. For them — and for the many who can't or won't take time — there is an effective medicine recently approved for prevention of AMS by the Federal Food and Drug Administration after being widely and successfully used for the last ten years. This is Diamox, or acetazolamide, a carbonic anhydrase inhibitor made by Lederle. That formidable descriptive name is important in understanding why and how it works.

Carbonic anhydrase (CAH) is an enzyme found almost everywhere in the body, but especially in red blood cells, kidneys, heart, and lungs. Its function is to catalyze the combination of carbon dioxide and water to bicarbonate, thus influencing the acidity or alkalinity of blood and also the excretion of bicarbonate in the urine. Chemicals that inhibit CAH do the following: (1) increase the tenacity with which red blood cells hold carbon dioxide, thus (2) decreasing the loss of carbon dioxide in the lung, thereby (3) decreasing alkalinity of blood, which (4) shifts the oxy-hemoglobin dissociation curve to the left, and thus (5) stimulates breathing slightly, while (6) increasing the flow of urine slightly. It is the combination of these actions that makes Diamox so valuable in preventing and even treating altitude illness. Stated simply: Diamox enables us to breathe more (thus getting more oxygen) without making the blood too alkaline, and to lose bicarbonate in urine, an important step in acclimatization.

But wait! In animals Diamox increases blood flow to the brain by 30 percent, though there's some argument over its effect in man. A recent study by Jack Reeves shows rather persuasively that the altitude headache is not related to increased cerebral blood flow. Why then should Diamox alleviate or prevent a headache that is unrelated to blood flow? More work is needed here.

We know that Diamox is a weak kidney stimulant (diuretic) for many people, and thus helps get rid of edema to a limited degree. But since many people do not experience this diuretic effect but do get relief, this explanation isn't enough. What we must be satisfied with at present is the fact that Diamox both relieves and prevents the altitude headache in most people, most of the time.

Recent work by Tom Johnson and Paul Rock at the Army Research Institute of Environmental Medicine, and by Peter Hackett and Robert Schoene on Mt. McKinley, indicate that dexamethasone, a member of the cortisone family, is also effective in preventing and treating AMS. The rationale for this effect is that dexamethasone reduces swelling of the brain, which some believe causes many of the symptoms of AMS.

But it is difficult to do controlled studies on a large enough number of people to be statistically significant, because not many people on vacation will agree to the possibility they might be given a placebo in the double-blind study required: "Doctor, I'm only here for a few days; give me the medicine that works." Experience with Diamox is growing even without large controlled studies (though some are in process as I write). One 250 mg tablet every six to eight hours — or the long-acting tablet every twelve hours — is an effective preventive or treatment.

Many other drugs have been tried over the years. Andean natives chew coca leaves, which probably help because of the small amount of cocaine they contain. Ammonium chloride was used for theoretically sound reasons but was rough on the stomach. A strong diuretic (furosemide) was considered beneficial by some but ineffective and dangerous by most others. Rolaids enjoyed brief notoriety until a carefully done study proved them no better than sugar pills. Aspirin has some special qualities which may make it effective; these are discussed in the chapter on HAPE.

As in so much of medicine, the placebo effect is strong. If the sufferer believes — or is persuasively told — that a medicine will help, it is likely to do so. "I did this and that happened" is an example of *post hoc, ergo propter hoc* ("after this, therefore because of this") reasoning, heard often in medicine, as in much of life! Unless and until a medication is carefully tested against an inactive substance, identical in appearance, under conditions where neither patient nor doctor knows medicine from placebo (the double-blind study), we cannot with certainty assess its value — and this is particularly true of AMS. Beware the placebo effect: it has led many doctors and patients astray.

Both theory and experimental evidence show that eating a diet high in carbohydrates is helpful, and we say that such a diet "lowers the altitude by 2,000 feet," which, of course, is a simplification. What happens is that a pure carbohydrate diet, where the ratio of carbon dioxide produced to oxygen consumed (the respiratory quotient RQ, or respiratory exchange ratio RE) is 1.0, allows the body to operate more efficiently than does a mixed diet, where the RQ is 0.7, and at altitude this is equivalent to being several thousand feet lower. Sugars, honey, jams, starches, and fruits are the best sources.

For several hours after any kind of meal, however, carbohydrates are the first substances metabolized, partly because they are more rapidly absorbed, partly because the body chooses quickly available fuel first. As a result, the respiratory quotient may be close to 1.0 for an hour or two even after an average, mixed meal. Later, when the ingested carbohydrates have been used, the fats and proteins in the meal are "burned" and the RQ falls. In practical terms this suggests that it's not necessary to eat only carbohydrates but that one should eat often. Small sweet or starchy meals every two or three hours will give the most altitude benefit. One must replace protein and fat because these are drawn from body stores when we don't eat. This is best done, not at night, because we don't want a low RQ during sleep when oxygen saturation is already lower than in the daytime, but on an off-day when not much work is to be done. The current wisdom for marathon runners (who push themselves as hard as high-altitude climbers) is to "load" carbohydrates for a few days before a demanding race; this may be good practice for mountaineers too.

Alcohol is a pure carbohydrate, but it has other effects which make it less suitable as a "food" at altitude: it impairs judgment and perception and other mental functions much as hypoxia does. It's likely to make you pass more water than you drink and thus may increase dehydration, and too much often leaves the indulgent with a hangover that is hard to distinguish from AMS. Alcohol is not a good food anywhere, especially in the mountains, and should be taken with discretion and appreciation.

Lots of experience and some theory indicate that drinking extra water is helpful, first because breathing so much dry air sucks water from the body when the saturated air is exhaled and this must be replaced. Second, dehydration thickens the blood, already beginning to thicken in response to hypoxia; thicker blood carries oxygen less efficiently and is more likely to form clots, so we want to avoid dehydration. Finally, we need to pass a lot of urine in order to eliminate bicarbonate (among other things), because lowering the blood bicarbonate is an important part of acclimatization. It may seem contradictory on the one hand to urge people to drink more water, while on the other hand we say that inability to handle water contributes to altitude illness. But altitude problems come from salt *and* water. Eating too much salt makes us hold water: we all know that after eating an especially salty meal, the water one thirsts for is retained and one can gain several pounds of "water weight" as a result. These are cogent arguments in favor of drinking a lot of water. Tea or coffee is also good, but too much caffeine is not conducive to sleep.

About exercise, experience and theory also agree: a little is helpful, too much or none is not. The responses stimulated by altitude are similar to those triggered by exertion: increased breathing (which better exchanges fresh for stale air deep in the lung), increased pulse rate and output of the heart (to move blood more rapidly about the body), opening of new capillaries (carrying oxygen to more cells), and diversion of blood from less to more demanding tissues. Moderate exertion increases the immediate responses to hypoxia; these may be overstressed by too much exertion, or not stimulated enough by bed rest. Stay on your feet, move about, but don't push yourself too hard for the first day or two at a new altitude.

Think positively! One thing that hard-core scientists have grudgingly come to acknowledge in recent years is the immense power of the spirit over the body. For decades doctors have recognized that mind and body react strongly to each other, but few were willing to accept that the mind can do so much to alter the physical body. Fear, anger, frustration harm many organs, perhaps every part of the body; joy, humor, satisfaction can heal. Laughter is as magical as sorrow is depressing. Meditation can relieve many problems both physical and emotional. Don't be afraid of high mountains: approach them with respect and admiration and try to draw from them relaxation and enjoyment of their marvelous beauty. Even without hard scientific data to support me, I am sure that one's mental state influences whether one is sick or well in the mountains.

AMS is usually more uncomfortable than threatening, it seldom needs any treatment, and its symptoms usually go away in a day or two. For the mild case, little more than patience is needed. Keep up and about, don't exercise too strenuously, eat lightly, and drink a lot of water. A pain reliever like aspirin or the equivalent may help the headache somewhat; codeine is more effective but seldom needed. Breathing oxygen does help, but symptoms return when oxygen is stopped. Getting down even a few thousand feet brings relief. More severe cases — especially if vomiting threatens to worsen dehydration — may require intravenous fluids to restore the depleted blood volume.

Remember that not everything which causes symptoms at altitude is due to AMS; one can as easily develop "flu" or some other infection, or food poisoning, or a hangover at altitude as at sea level. If in doubt, get some informed medical care.

AMS is not an inevitable feature of mountain travel: it is

preventable and treatable. It need not spoil a planned vacation or an expensive mountain trek halfway around the world. Too many tourists on ill-designed tours to Machu Picchu, Kilimanjaro, or Everest Base Camp, and too many skiers visiting thousands of ski resorts here and abroad have had their enjoyment tarnished, or gone home ill from this avoidable unpleasantness.

It doesn't have to happen to you!

Chapter Ten

HIGH-ALTITUDE PULMONARY EDEMA (HAPE)

TWO OF THE WORKMEN who built Angelo Mosso's laboratory on Monte Rosa developed congestion of the lungs that might have been pneumonia. But Mosso was aware of other possibilities and quoted from an account of a tragedy on Mont Blanc written by Dr. Guglielminetti a few years previously. The victim, a young physician named Jacottet, had joined a rescue party despite "mild indisposition" a few days earlier. The scene was the Vallot hut at 14,300 feet:

On the first of September, after a day's rest in the hut, during which Jacottet seemed to feel better than he did at first, he climbed to the summit, remained there an hour, and then returned to the hut. During the night he did not sleep and coughed much, and complained at breakfast of headache and lack of appetite. During the morning he wrote a letter to his brother at Vienne, in which he remarked that he had passed so bad a night that he did not wish the like to his worst enemy. His distress increased to such a degree that Imfeld advised him to descend to Chamonix, but he refused. He wrote another letter to one of his friends, telling him that he could not write at greater length because of the sick feeling which was tormenting him, that he was suffering from mountain sickness like the others, but that he meant to study the influence of atmospheric depression and acclimatize himself. This alas was his last letter! He afterwards threw himself on his bed trembling with cold. On the 2nd September . . . he seemed as para-

lyzed and began to wander. Oxygen was given him to breathe but without result. The respiration was superficial (60 to 70 breaths per minute), the pulse irregular (between 100 and 120), the temperature 38.3 degrees C. Towards six o'clock in the evening he suddenly ceased to speak, became somnolent, and then the death agony began. His face grew pale, and towards 2 A.M. he expired in the glacier hut, a victim of his devotion to science, like a soldier on a battlefield.

From Dr. Wizard's post-mortem examination it appeared that Dr. Jacottet had died of capillary bronchitis and lobular pneumonitis. The immediate cause of death was therefore probably a suffocative catarrh, accompanied by acute edema of the lung.

These diagnoses are not used today and may have indicated some form of pneumonia. Pulmonary edema from heart failure was well known, but there was no reason to suspect this in such a healthy young man. Heart disease was not mentioned in another account of the episode written by a leading Swiss physician, Dr. Egli-Sinclair, who blamed the death on *"mal de montagne."* I have not been able to find the autopsy report, but the cause of death is listed as "congestion of the lungs" in the records of the town clerk in Chamonix.

Dr. Ravenhill, describing his experience in a mining camp at 15,000 feet in Peru, described several cases that are even more characteristic of HAPE:

An Englishman, Mr. V—— ... arrived in the usual way, by train — a forty-two-hour journey from sea level.... He seemed in good health on arrival, and said that he felt quite well, but nevertheless he kept quiet, ate sparingly and went to bed early. He woke next morning feeling ill with symptoms of the normal type of puna. *As the day drew on he began to feel very ill indeed.... He became very cyanosed, had evident air hunger.... He seemed to present the typical picture of a failing heart. This condition persisted during the night; he coughed up with difficulty. He vomited at intervals. He had several inhalations of oxygen; strychnine and digitalis were also given. Towards morning he recovered slightly and as there was luckily a train ... he was sent straight down.... I heard that when he got down to 12,000*

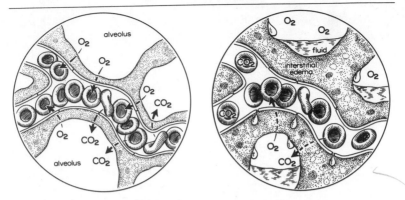

FIGURE 28. NORMAL AND FLUID-FILLED ALVEOLI

Normally the tiny alveoli, though moist, contain no free fluid, and the thin membrane which separates each from its surrounding capillary network is little more than two molecular faces (*left*). Carbon dioxide and oxygen pass freely through the membrane with little or no drop in pressure. However, when edema begins to form (from heart failure or from oxygen lack), it appears first between the capillary wall and the alveolus, thus increasing the pressure drop between alveolar oxygen and that in blood. Carbon dioxide, diffusing more readily, is less affected. As the condition worsens (*right*), fluid seeps through the alveolar membrane into the alveoli, where its presence can be detected by gurgles and crackles heard during breathing. The victim tries to cough up this liquid and often raises large amounts of thin, frothy fluid which usually becomes pink or even bloody. As the fluid increases, it is more and more difficult for oxygen to enter the blood, and the patient begins to drown in his own fluids.

feet he was considerably better and at 7,000 feet he was nearly well. It seemed to me that he would have died had he stayed in the altitude for another day.

This is a clear and accurate description of a typical case of HAPE: symptoms gradually developing after rapid ascent, growing worse in a few hours with signs of moisture in the lungs, and, after threatening to be fatal, improving rapidly during descent. Today we know that HAPE is not due to a failing heart, as Ravenhill evidently believed when he called it "cardiac *puna.*"

In 1937 Alberto Hurtado, who would become one of the world authorities in high-altitude illness, was inducted into the National Academy of Medicine in Lima, offering as his thesis a long paper titled "Pathology of Life at High Altitude." In it he described five cases of mountain sickness, giving more laboratory and X-ray evidence than had previously been obtained. Four of his cases resemble subacute or chronic mountain sickness, but the fifth was either an unusual form of high-altitude pulmonary edema or heart failure.

Man, 58 years old . . . of Indian race. During the last 29 years he has lived in area of high elevation. He has been in Lima on various occasions and never has had Soroche upon returning. . . . After being in Lima for three days he returned to Oroya by train. At . . . 13,000 feet he feels extremely badly, he begins to cough and he observes that his saliva contains a great deal of black blood. Soon there was added to his symptoms: headache, intense difficulty in respiration and a certain mental incoordination. . . . At the examination he presents: Orthopnea, very intense cyanosis, expression of anxiety . . . and crepitant rales over both lungs. Expectoration is typically abundant, red and foamy (contains blood). An X-ray of the thorax shows an evident diminution of the pulmonary transparency. . . . Taken down to Lima the patient improves slowly and after two months he ascends again. A detailed examination at this time reveals the signs of circulatory insufficiency (congestion at the base of the lungs and edema of the extremities). However this time he does not show acute congestion.

Few of those who quote Hurtado have read this hard-to-find paper, and this case, the one most suggestive of HAPE, might be attributed to another cause, such as congestive heart failure or pulmonary embolism. Today, because of easy and rapid access to many places high enough to be dangerous, characteristic cases are more common:

A fifty-two-year-old man flew from Pittsburgh to Denver and drove at once to 9,000 feet. Next day he saw a doctor because of severe headache, inability to sleep, lethargy, shortness of breath, and scanty urination. On examination he looked poorly, had scattered moisture in both lungs but no other abnormalities. Chest X ray was typical of HAPE; he was given oxygen for a short time with benefit, and then drove down to 5,000 feet and was completely recovered on arrival.

This is a more common scenario, which unfortunately has been played out hundreds of times in recent years. It probably happened many times in the past but went unrecognized for what it is now known to be: an accumulation of fluid in the lungs caused by lack of oxygen. Though this is most commonly due to altitude, we know that lack of oxygen rather than decreased atmospheric pressure is the cause: aviators and mountaineers can go very high without risk of edema if they breathe oxygen. At sea level other conditions that cause hypoxia can produce pulmonary edema indistinguishable from that seen in the mountains.

Hurtado's privately printed thesis went unnoticed for thirty years while a number of strong young climbers died as Dr. Jacottet did. A description of the final days of one brilliant climber, who died two years before HAPE became widely recognized, has since been widely quoted:

Over a five-day period W.B. climbed to 16,000 feet with a heavy pack. He was far more short of breath than others in the party, did not eat, and began to cough. A companion later said that "he obviously had fluid in his lungs." Despite penicillin his breathing rapidly became more labored, his cough more severe and frequent, and as his companion wrote in his diary: "Over the next hours W.B.'s breathing became progressively more congested and labored. He sounded as though he were literally drowning in his own fluid with an almost continuous loud bubbling noise as if breathing through liquid." His breathing grew far worse during the night, he became limp, and died at dawn on the second day of illness.

In 1958 I was involved in an episode that seemed unimportant at the time but has since had large consequences:

On December 28, 1958, two healthy college students crossed a 12,000-foot pass where one of them developed severe shortness of

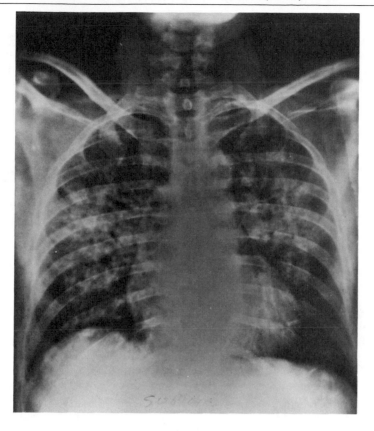

*FIGURE 29. A TYPICAL CASE OF HIGH-ALTITUDE
PULMONARY EDEMA*

This X-ray photograph is characteristic of HAPE except that the patient was stricken at only 9,500 feet, whereas HAPE usually occurs at a somewhat higher altitude. The neck shadow at the top and the dense dome of the diaphragm at the bottom are easily identified. In the center of the picture is the flask-shaped shadow of the heart, protruding more toward the right of the photograph (left ventricle). The curved white lines on each side are ribs, and the darker areas represent air-filled lung tissue, which easily transmits the X-ray beam. Scattered throughout both lungs, though more in the right one, are fluffy white patches which represent something denser than lung tissue, and in this case are caused by accumulations of fluid.

breath, weakness, and cough. They descended slowly, but over the next thirty-six hours his symptoms became so severe that he could not go on, and his companion left him in a tent and went for help. Early in the evening of the thirty-first he reached me, and after several hours of trying to muster a reasonably sober rescue party, we set off at dawn on January 1, reaching the boy about noon and bringing him out to the hospital; my tentative diagnosis was pneumonia. A careful work-up showed pulmonary edema with no obvious explanation, and he recovered rapidly.

When it became clear that this was not a simple case of pneumonia but of pulmonary edema, usually associated with heart failure, I referred him to a heart specialist, who concluded that the boy must have some form of heart disease, despite the absence of any other evidence. The matter might have ended there, but my good friend Dr. Paul Dudley White, a distinguished cardiologist, happened to be visiting me, reviewed the story, and said it was not heart disease but somehow related to altitude and should be published.

In an article that appeared in the *New England Journal of Medicine* reporting this case and several similar ones that had been described to me by climbing friends, I proposed that this was an affliction due to altitude and breathing cold air and not heart failure; I was soon deluged with letters from around the world describing similar cases. I did not know until later that Dr. Herbert Hultgren had been studying a number of such cases in South America and would soon publish a more complete description of HAPE — as it by then had become known — a reversible, potentially fatal derangement of fluid balance in the lung caused by too rapid ascent to high altitude. Time has shown that from 0.05 to 1.0 percent of all who go above 9,000 feet taking too little time to adjust will be victims of HAPE and one out of ten of these will die of this avoidable disturbance.

Once HAPE was recognized as due to altitude hypoxia and

not to preexisting heart or lung disease, the question of why such changes should occur became important. We already knew that blood pressure in the pulmonary artery is increased at altitude and in fact by hypoxia of any cause. (The pulmonary artery carries blood returning from all parts of the body through the heart to the lungs, where it picks up oxygen and returns to the heart. It is the only artery that carries venous blood, that is, blood depleted of oxygen.) So far as we knew, the higher the altitude or the more severe the hypoxia caused by illness, the higher the pulmonary artery pressure (PAP). This was especially interesting because blood pressure in the systemic circulation (which supplies the rest of the body) increases only slightly if at all at altitude.

One possibility was that breathing cold air might cause constriction of the smaller vessels in the lungs — just as cold constricts the blood vessels in the skin — and thus might raise PAP. This explanation seemed unlikely after Ben Eiseman and others showed that even extremely cold air was warmed to body temperature before it reached the lungs. But that idea was revived recently when John Bligh and his associates found what appears to be a reflex originating inside the nostrils that responds to cold air by increasing the pressure in the pulmonary artery! Just how important this may be in HAPE needs to be studied — and we must remember that HAPE can and does occur in warm weather too.

During the next decade, important observations were made in many parts of the world, although some were more puzzling than helpful. It was found that PAP increased within minutes of exposure to low oxygen and returned to normal as soon as normal oxygen was restored. This suggested temporary spasm of the pulmonary arteries and increased pulmonary resistance. No evidence of heart failure or increased pressure in any of the chambers of the heart was found.

PAP increased sharply during exercise, often going higher than it did at altitude, but edema of the lungs seldom resulted

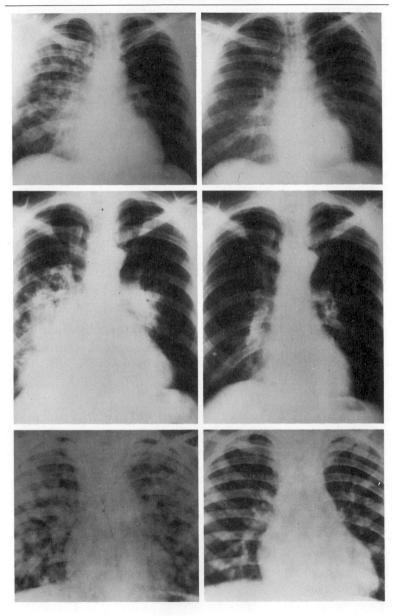

FIGURE 30. VARIOUS FORMS OF HIGH-ALTITUDE PULMONARY EDEMA

As these three pairs of X-ray photographs show, high-altitude pulmonary edema (HAPE) can take several forms.

Top row: This thirty-five-year-old physician was mistakenly diagnosed as having an asthmatic attack when he became very short of breath at a ski resort at 8,000 feet and his doctor heard wheezes and wet crackles in his chest. The X ray taken when he was admitted to the hospital (*left*) shows fluffy white shadows scattered throughout the right lung, while the left lung seems to be almost completely normal. Three days later (*right*), both lungs have cleared and transmit the X-ray beam well because the lungs are again filled with air, leaving only the central heart shadow and the ribs to interfere with passage of X rays.

Middle row: This young skier became very short of breath and weak while crossing a 12,000-foot pass, but managed to get down to 9,000 feet where he was later rescued. When he reached the hospital, an X ray (*left*) showed dense shadows at the "root" of each lung (close to the heart), which could be due to many things. Two days later (*right*), all but small normal shadows have disappeared, strongly suggesting (together with the examination and laboratory findings) that the shadows were due to fluid (HAPE). This patient, being tall and thin, has a narrow, long chest and a narrow "vertical" heart.

Bottom row: This traveler became very short of breath and obviously extremely ill at 14,000 feet. The first X ray (*left*) shows white fluffy shadows scattered everywhere in both lungs almost obscuring the normal rib and heart shadows. Only one day later (*right*), both lungs are almost completely clear; the shadows of fluid patches have almost disappeared, although here and there (especially in the upper outer part of the left lung) some fluid still can be seen.

These pictures show how variable the X ray can be and how rapidly the shadows caused by fluid can disappear. From the variety of forms HAPE takes, it is not surprising that it is (or used to be) often mistaken for pneumonia or some other serious medical condition.

---

except after very strenuous exertion, such as the Comrades ninety-kilometer marathon in South Africa, where several cases of pulmonary edema occur each year, although the run is not at high altitude.

The elevated PAP found in visitors and short-term residents

stayed high while at altitude, but fell to normal on return to sea level. The PAP of some races of altitude natives was high, but in others it was normal. Those with high PAP were found to have thick-walled pulmonary arterioles, which was also true of persons with diseases that made them chronically hypoxic at sea level. The PAP of such individuals did not return to normal when oxygen was given.

Many animals showed a sharp increase in PAP when taken to altitude, but others did not. Some animals native to high altitude, like the llama and vicuna, had normal pulmonary artery pressures and no thickening of the muscle layers of the pulmonary vessels, but other animals, like the yak, had both high pressure and thick-walled vessels.

The X-ray picture of HAPE was quite different from that seen in other forms of pulmonary edema, such as heart failure. HAPE looks as though many snowballs were scattered through one or both lungs (more often in the right) and is easily recognized, or should be. The X ray suggests that edema occurs here and there at random. We needed to know what the fluid was, where it came from, and why it was so randomly distributed. It is not easy to get samples of fluid from deep in the lung: what is coughed up in HAPE is mixed with saliva.

Rob Schoene and Peter Hackett, working at 14,000 feet on Mt. McKinley, were seeing several severe cases of HAPE each year and bravely inserted a flexible bronchoscope deep in the lungs of several patients, drew out fluid from the alveoli, and showed that it was much like plasma (the liquid portion of blood). This meant it must have leaked through the walls of the blood vessels into the alveoli. The question then became why fluid should leak in some places and not in others, if the pressure in the vessels (which presumably drove the leakage) was the same everywhere in the lungs.

Hultgren had been suggesting for many years that blood flow was not the same everywhere, but that some parts of the lungs received more blood under higher pressure than others; these areas would leak, he thought. Gary Gray, who knew that divers develop tiny bubbles in their blood (much like those that form when a bottle of soda is uncapped) when coming rapidly from the high pressure of a dive to normal pressure at sea level, transferred this observation to mountaineers. Knowing that aviators going too high too fast sometimes developed pain similar to the bends seen in divers, Gray proposed that mountaineers too might have little bubbles in the blood that might persist even during a comparatively slow climb and suggested that perhaps blood platelets collected around these micro-bubbles and lodged in the capillaries of the lung, causing patches of obstruction here and there. By injecting platelets tagged with radioactive chromium into subjects then taken to altitude in a decompression chamber and X-rayed, he showed that small migrating "clots" called microemboli did in fact land randomly in the lungs.

The "bubble" idea has been extensively studied at Shinshu University in Japan, where Kobayashi, Ueda, Levine, and others have done a series of elegant studies on sheep. Delicate catheters were placed in the major duct carrying lymph from the lungs in order to measure changes in fluid accumulation in lung tissue, and in the heart and pulmonary artery to measure blood flow and pressure. After the animals recovered completely, one group was taken slowly to altitude (in a decompression chamber) breathing sea level oxygen; a second group was kept at sea level pressure but breathed low oxygen; while a third group was taken to altitude breathing air. Measurements were made during a two-hour stay at each of three simulated altitudes: 8,500 feet, 15,000 feet, and 21,500 feet. Lymph flow increased significantly only when the sheep were exposed to both low pressure and low oxygen; neither low pressure nor low oxygen alone caused a change. They concluded that microscopic air bubbles contributed to the accumulation of fluid and thus were a factor in HAPE.

Now sheep are different from humans, and the protocols used by the Japanese, like those used by Staub and others before, may not apply to man. Nevertheless, until we have better understanding of the mechanisms, it is possible that micro-bubbles contribute to the ventilation–perfusion mismatch postulated by Hultgren and Gray and actually measured by Peter Wagner and others.

Further support came from studies of an interesting substance called surfactant, which thinly coats the lining of the lower respiratory passages. This increases surface tension in the alveoli, which would otherwise collapse inward. The smaller the sphere, the greater its tendency to collapse. Surfactant is constantly being made and destroyed in the lungs, and hypoxia interferes with its production. We know that when surfactant is decreased by disease or infection, patches of alveoli collapse. It may be that altitude hypoxia, by diminishing surfactant, causes this kind of collapse, so that parts of the lungs receive enough blood but not enough air.

Might a combination of these responses cause some people to develop mild pulmonary edema, so subtle that it would cause few or no symptoms? There is more and more indication that many — possibly most — people do accumulate traces of fluid in the loose interstitial space during their first few days at altitude. In most people the circulation of the lung is able to absorb this fluid as fast as it forms, but in others fluid builds up and HAPE results.

An unusual case provided some important evidence supporting Hultgren's old theory in March 1975 when Miriam VanHardenbroeck consulted me about an unfortunate young soldier:

M.P. was a healthy twenty-nine-year-old man who came rapidly from Missouri to 9,500 feet. He skied for a few hours but sprained his ankle and sat around the lodge for the rest of the day. Cough and shortness of breath began in the afternoon and worsened during the night and next day he began to vomit, and to cough more. By the end of the afternoon he was very ill, and died as he was being driven to see a doctor. Postmortem X ray showed extensive pulmonary edema; autopsy showed that he had been born with no major artery to one lung (congenital absence of a pulmonary artery).

Though this was an interesting and unusual condition, its coincidence with HAPE meant little, but three months later VanHardenbroeck called again. She had just seen a second patient with severe HAPE: this lady was more fortunate, for she recovered after being sent to a hospital at lower altitude, where she was found to have the same condition — absence of one pulmonary artery.

Now this is a rare birth defect and the chances of the two people also getting unusually severe HAPE by coincidence were small. It was far more likely that the abnormality was a clue to a fundamental cause of HAPE. I reported these cases at several medical meetings, and within a year heard of others which Peter Hackett and colleagues tracked down and published. Since then several more individuals have turned up who are affected at a low enough altitude to present an extra problem:

In 1981, C.C. went on vacation with his family in the Sierras. On reaching 7,000 feet he complained of chest pain, difficulty sleeping, and headache. Next day after a short bicycle ride he was very tired and began to cough and bring up a lot of sputum during the night. His mother and his physician-grandfather felt he might have HAPE and started for sea level. An hour later at 5,000 feet a chest X ray proved that he did have HAPE; he recovered promptly as he was taken to sea level. Five years previously, absence of one pulmonary artery had been diagnosed, but the risk of going to altitude was not appreciated at that time.

I now know of ten persons with this birth defect who have developed severe HAPE at moderate altitude, one or two as low as 5,000 feet. These cases add support to the ventilation–perfusion mismatch theory because we believe that altitude, by increasing pulmonary artery pressure in the already overperfused lung, triggers edema and makes it especially dangerous. Such people may even be at risk if they fly for more than a few hours, since commercial aircraft are generally pressurized to a cabin altitude of 5,000 to 7,500 feet.

Meanwhile, other groups were studying patients who had

high blood pressure in the pulmonary arteries at sea level for no apparent reason, and some whose pressure was high because they had a disease that caused lack of oxygen. They found that several powerful substances were released in the lungs when blood pressure and flow were high, stretching the vessels. Some of these caused small blood vessels (arterioles) to contract, but others caused them to dilate. Still other substances caused blood platelets to clump, while their antagonists prevented clumping. To further complicate the picture, some of these platelet-activating substances, released when pulmonary blood pressure and flow are high, caused nearby capillaries to leak.

It now looks as though the development of high-altitude edema depends on which one of each of these pairs of antagonists prevails. If the constrictors and the platelet clumpers and the leak makers are stronger than their opposites, edema may appear; otherwise not. This would depend on certain characteristics of the individual (now unknown) as well as on the condition of different parts of the lung.

Assuming that these observations stand the test of time, we may now write a better description of how HAPE develops. Based on what we know and what we can reasonably extrapolate, it could run like this:

1. Hypoxia from whatever cause immediately increases pulmonary artery pressure and blood flow, both of which are further increased by exercise.
2. Increased pulmonary blood pressure and flow stretch the vessels and are associated with release of substances that act on the blood vessels and on the circulating platelets. This allows fluid to leak from the capillaries.
3. At first the fluid is reabsorbed as rapidly as it is formed, but as seepage increases, edema fluid accumulates between the wall of the alveolus and the blood vessel (called the interstitial space), distending it and then leaking into the alveoli.

4. Platelets form small clumps when there is an imbalance between the substances released from cells in the capillary walls and in the blood, and possibly around minute bubbles caused by decompression. The resulting tiny clots (microemboli) obstruct small vessels in the lung, diverting blood flow to other parts of the lung. Differences in the tone of the small vessels and imbalance between the opposing effects of the different substances released cause further changes in circulation in scattered parts of the lungs, flooding some and leaving others poorly perfused.

5. The increasing mismatch between ventilation and perfusion plus the stretching of blood vessels tends to shear the lining of the capillaries and opens the junctions, normally tight, between cells. The shear forces release more active substances and further stretch the vessels. These widened gaps allow red cells to leave the capillaries and to enter the alveoli along with plasma.

6. As fluid accumulates in some of the interstitial spaces, it impedes the passage of oxygen from those alveoli to their capillary net, thus further increasing the overall mismatch between ventilation and perfusion, and the whole process accelerates.

In summary then, high-altitude pulmonary edema appears to have elements of both high pressure and high permeability edema — high pressure on the arterial side, and high permeability (leakiness) in the capillaries of the lung. There is also some inequality between ventilation and perfusion, that is, some areas have good blood flow but are poorly aerated, while in other areas the reverse is true. Whether this is due to small microemboli or clumps of platelets, to collapse of small areas caused by breakdown of surfactant, or to local spasm of small vessels is unclear. We don't understand why some individuals have repeated attacks of pulmonary edema while others, taking greater risks, do not. We don't know why altitude residents who return after a short stay at sea level should be more susceptible, if indeed they are. We don't know how or why pulmonary artery pressure is increased immediately after exposure to hypoxia of any type. It may be due to signals from the brain (the "central theory"), or to increased secretion of one of the powerful hormones which are known to be stimulated by hypoxia, or to a combination of both. The patchy nature of the edema suggests that local changes, such as narrowing of small vessels, are due to substances released locally.

The best management for HAPE is to get down. Descent of only a few thousand feet usually brings dramatic improvement, so much that a few patients, unconscious when air-lifted from a mountain, have even complained on arrival at low altitude that evacuation was unnecessary — and refused to pay! Mild early cases will often respond to oxygen and rest, and this is safe providing the patient can have hospital care and all that goes with it. On a mountain expedition, getting down should be mandatory as soon as it is clear the patient has HAPE. It is too dangerous to "wait and see if the medicine (or oxygen) works": a storm may come up, the victim may soon be unable to walk or may rapidly lose consciousness. Oxygen does help, but not as much as getting down.

Occasionally — though rarely — getting down isn't effective. In fact, in the first case I ever saw, descending 3,000 feet did not help at all. Here's a case of HAPE that developed very rapidly while descending after a 5,300-foot climb to 20,300 feet. The patient is an unusually strong, fast climber, a practicing physician-anesthesiologist, and an astute observer.

The party took two weeks to walk from 2,500 to 12,000 feet and in the next two days reached 15,000 feet without difficulty. Next day she and three others climbed a rather easy 20,300-foot peak some three to four miles distant, reaching the top late in the day feeling very well. They then descended 1,500 feet rapidly, but were delayed and felt the cold. Then on a long easy walk, as she wrote later: "Suddenly I couldn't keep up. . . . I was exhausted but also very short of breath. I couldn't get enough air. . . . I developed very severe pain in my chest

*... and at times had to stop walking because of pain. ... I thought of
a pulmonary embolus. I had no headache at any time. Balance was
difficult. After a time walking down the glacier I had to stop every few
steps to breathe. ... I kept taking an occasional step until we reached
camp, though I was thoroughly convinced I would never make it and
was going to die." She sat up all night; the pain soon disappeared but
she had trouble breathing and her pulse was too fast to count. She was
aware of gurgling in her chest. She felt as though she had grippe, but
after a day of sleep she was able to climb over a low pass and went
home, improving steadily. It is interesting that she had been taking
three Diamox tablets daily for two days. She recovered completely.*

This was undoubtedly a severe case of HAPE, which could
have been fatal in a less capable, less knowledgeable individual. Why it did not start until she had descended 1,500 feet is
not explained; cold may have had some effect.

Usually getting down brings improvement swiftly and dramatically. One might therefore expect that increasing pressure
in the lungs might also help. Several apparatuses that do this
have been beneficial when used in hospitals. On an expedition
these are not available, but a large bag (with windows to see
through) in which the victim is placed and the bag then inflated to whatever pressure is desired is being tested. A coffin-
like box has already been used as a small pressure chamber:
the patient lies inside, the lid is tightly closed, and a pump increases the pressure in the box. A Japanese team working at
Pheriche near Everest reports that thirty minutes in this "com-
pression box" with an inside pressure equal to that at 5,200 feet
produces rapid improvement.

More practical may be a snug-fitting mask that covers mouth
and nose. The wearer breathes in without difficulty through a
valve that is slightly spring-loaded so that he exhales against
some resistance, thus increasing pressure in his lungs. This also
helps to reexpand small areas in the lung that have col-
lapsed — not uncommon in HAPE. The device is light, inex-
pensive, and easy to carry. Preliminary tests have shown that it
increases oxygen in the blood — and helps to retain carbon

dioxide, which may be more important — but the device needs to be used in more cases before we will know how helpful it is. Breathing out against pursed lips ("grunt breathing") has a certain vogue with some, but it is difficult and no more beneficial than deliberately increasing breathing slightly. Overbreathing was used as an emergency measure in World War II when aircrew lost their oxygen supplies at altitude: this enabled men to survive long enough to reach safety.

Diamox is being used more and more to treat both AMS and HAPE; larger or more frequent doses may be needed to take advantage of the diuretic action as well as its inhibition of carbonic anhydrase. So far no controlled studies have been done, but an increasing number of stories proclaim its value, and it sounds logical and safe.

Furosemide (Lasix) is a more powerful diuretic — too powerful sometimes. In early cases of HAPE it can "squeeze water out of the lungs" and produce a copious flow of urine, rapidly clearing the lungs. But sometimes urination is so copious that the patient may go into shock due to decreased blood volume (called hypovolemic shock). Thus one may risk converting a sick but walking victim to a litter case. Paradoxical though it may seem, if water is poured in one end as fast as it is lost at the other, furosemide is effective treatment for pulmonary edema. Furosemide given intravenously also lowers pulmonary artery pressure, which is helpful.

Morphine is often valuable in pulmonary edema due to heart failure, but it has not been used often in HAPE for fear of depressing breathing. Digitalis and other excellent cardiac drugs are of no value whatever in HAPE, because the heart is normal. For the same reason, putting tourniquets around the legs, or drawing off blood — both old-fashioned treatments for acute heart failure — are of no value and may actually make matters worse. Similarly, drugs used to control asthma (like aminophylline and its cousins) are useless.

Since high pulmonary artery pressure contributes strongly to HAPE, a medication that lowers this pressure by dilating the small vessels in the lung would seem a logical treatment. This type of drug is being studied now and shows promise but will have to be tested under controlled conditions before being recommended for use in the field.

HAPE is potentially so dangerous that getting down if one can do so is better and safer than staying in bed at altitude and breathing oxygen. At the same time, it is reasonable to hold a patient at altitude if he can be cared for in a good hospital and evacuated immediately if he shows signs of getting worse. Obviously oxygen should be given to the climber who cannot get down because of a storm or other reason, and it may reverse the process.

Not surprisingly, some gung-ho mountaineer, stricken with HAPE and evacuated, may improve so much that he insists on returning to finish his climb. Sometimes he may pull it off: Robert Roach tells me that two of eleven HAPE victims evacuated from high on McKinley recovered so completely that they returned and climbed to the summit with no recurrence. Those are not good odds, when you realize the risks and effort expended to rescue a victim. More often we see the following scenario, relayed to me by David Shlim:

An experienced mountaineer developed what sounds like HAPE and HACE after going too fast to 17,500 feet in the Everest region. He had enough sense to start down the valley, and almost made it to safety before collapsing. Another party helped him to Pheriche, where he was treated in the Japanese pressure box and felt much better. He was told he might go back up after a few days, which he did, slowly. Once he had arrived at his base camp (about 19,000 feet), he decided to solo the mountain and climbed a very steep pitch before settling down in his hammock slung from the rocks. He woke at midnight very sick, and descended, semiconscious, alone. Fortunately he was found and again treated in the pressure box, and managed to walk down for three days and was flown to Kathmandu, where he was completely well.

One can only shudder at the risks taken by this individual and the trouble he caused for others. There have been other less extreme examples of recurrence during reascent, and it is not a very good idea!

Every year brings better understanding of this "physiological illness" that affects the young, the bold, and the healthy, as Drummond Rennie pointed out, because these are — or have been — the ones most at risk. But more and more people of all ages and different health are going to the mountains to work or to play, so it is as important to teach them about altitude as to provide them with drugs.

As for all altitude illnesses, the best prevention is to take time — time to relax and enjoy the mountains, time to let the body make its adjustments. How fast is slow enough? Above 5,000 feet, allow one day for each additional 1,000 feet is the usual advice, but it is probably more appropriate to go up a bit faster and to sleep at an altitude lower than where one spends each day. Diamox may prevent, or at least decrease, the risk of HAPE as well as AMS, but we should not rely on medication to do the job that Nature does so much better. Drink lots of water, take little salt or alcohol, increase exertion gradually. And above all, start down if HAPE develops.

Finally we must look at a familiar medicine: aspirin. After more than a century of extensive use, we do not know exactly how this remarkable drug affects a large family of natural body products — the prostaglandins, found in almost every type of tissue, and probably involved in HAPE. Aspirin prevents the clumping (aggregation) of platelets, and therefore, if platelet aggregation is a factor in HAPE, aspirin could logically be expected to have some preventive action, just as it may have in preventing blockage of blood vessels in the heart muscle. Should we therefore take an aspirin every day at altitude? Though I certainly wouldn't advise this routinely, it may be reasonable, though we must not forget that aspirin has bad effects on some people who are sensitive to it or who may develop gastric irritation and even bleeding.

Those who have had HAPE once are probably at greater risk

for recurrence, though why this should be we do not know (assuming there are none of the underlying problems mentioned above). Someone who has had several attacks should look for a different recreation, but since he probably will not, he should definitely climb much more slowly — and probably take Diamox before and during the climb.

It's generally believed that children under five or six are more vulnerable to HAPE, but the evidence for this is not firm, and a recent study seems to indicate that they are no more or less susceptible than adults. The elderly are no more likely than anyone else to have HAPE. So the best evidence today is that age plays little or no part in high-altitude pulmonary edema.

Persons living at 8,000 feet and above may develop HAPE when they return after a brief stay at sea level. This is not proven, but the evidence is piling up. Many thousands of people live at such altitudes and most of them go down to low altitude now and then for short or long stays. If HAPE were much more common under such conditions, I believe we would have heard much more about it. Nevertheless, altitude residents should take more time to return to altitude and be more watchful for symptoms — and perhaps take Diamox!

Over the years we have come to recognize that a respiratory infection, even a mild cold or bronchitis, seems to increase the likelihood of HAPE. Why this should be so we do not know. But today I advise those with fresh respiratory infections either to delay an ascent or to be especially watchful.

Obviously persons known to have an absent pulmonary artery or a history of pulmonary embolus or loss of all or part of a lung need to be carefully advised before going to even moderate altitude.

From a historical viewpoint it is interesting that the Director General of the Indian Armed Forces Medical Services, on October 20, 1962 (during the heat of the "boundary conflict" with China), issued a small booklet containing the following orders:

. . . Previously acclimatized individuals of high altitude areas, returning to altitude after leave, and individuals who have had a previous attack should be aware of the possibility of acute high altitude pulmonary oedema whenever they are involved in a rapid ascent to an altitude in excess of 9,000 feet.

. . . Gradual acclimatization should be observed.

. . . Undue physical exertion at high altitude should be avoided during the first 48 hours after arrival.

. . . Persons suffering from viral infection should not make trips to high altitude.

It would be difficult today to improve significantly on these orders, written only a year after publication of the first descriptions of HAPE.

Chapter Eleven

HIGH-ALTITUDE CEREBRAL EDEMA (HACE)

LACK OF OXYGEN affects the higher centers of the brain subtly at first but occasionally the impact may be devastating. One need not go very high to get into bad trouble, which can be aggravated by failure to appreciate just what is happening:

Bill drove from New York to 8,400 in Wyoming and a day later set off on a cross-country ski trip as he had done before. Each day the party struggled through deep snow, climbing only a few hundred feet; each day Bill's headache grew worse and he had more difficulty keeping up and fell a lot. On the fifth day (at 10,500 feet) he was near collapse, and next morning when rescue arrived he was deeply unconscious and rigid. In the hospital an X ray showed pulmonary edema and a neurological examination was abnormal. He improved slowly, regaining consciousness in forty-eight hours, though mumbling and irrational; after four days he was almost well. He recalls "seeing Marilyn Monroe, live and in color, on the hospital walls" until the day he left.

Bill almost died because he and his companions simply didn't realize how serious hypoxia can be even at relatively low altitude and a slow rate of climb. If they had turned back a few days earlier, he would probably have recovered easily, but a day later he might have died.

A thirty-eight-year-old man went to bed asking not to be disturbed, soon after driving to 12,000 feet from sea level. Twenty-four hours later he could not be roused and was in deep coma, with rigid arms and legs, weak pulse, dilated pupils, and evidence of pulmonary edema. Though hospitalized and intensively treated, he died.

For years we have used the term "high-altitude cerebral edema" or HACE to describe this kind of neurological altitude illness, which Ravenhill called "nervous *puna*." But is this designation accurate or appropriate? Does the brain really develop edema and swell? Is there a distinctive entity deserving this or some similar name where only the brain is affected? Or does oxygen lack affect the brain in *all* forms of altitude illness? Should we consider instead, as John Dickinson does, a name like "cerebral acute mountain sickness" (CAMS)? We can answer such questions only approximately today, influenced by our individual biases. The term HACE may be imprecise (as are many other words we use in medicine), but it is a convenient way to describe those cases of altitude illness where neurological signs and symptoms are the most prominent. Some prefer "high-altitude encephalopathy" (HAE), since this does not prejudge that the brain is actually swollen with fluid. I use HACE as shorthand to mean altitude illness affecting the brain more obviously than other organs.

Our brain is wrapped in delicate membranes, but unlike other organs it is cushioned in fluid within a rigid box which it completely fills. Since the skull has few openings, any increase in the size of the brain causes pressure throughout. Brain tissue feels no pain if injured, but the membranes which wrap it are extremely sensitive, as is the network of blood vessels which brings nutrients and oxygen and carries away carbon dioxide and other wastes.

When the brain is deprived of its normal oxygen supply, its large and small arteries dilate and the amount of blood they contain increases. Stretching their walls causes pain, and this contributes to altitude headache. Autopsies done on victims of HACE have shown that the brain, like other parts of the body, can and does swell when deprived of oxygen, presumably due to failure of the sodium pump. This swelling, together with the distended blood vessels, increases the volume of the brain and stretches the delicate films that cover it. In a few patients, the pressure of the spinal fluid that bathes the brain has been measured and found higher than normal, confirming the impression that the skull is overfilled. This has led us to believe that altitude headache is due to edema in and between brain cells, which causes stretching of the membranes that cover the brain and those that cover the engorged and distended blood vessels. This is a neat but simplistic explanation, and Jack Reeves for one does not believe that increased blood flow explains altitude headache. Much more work is needed here.

Since virtually all activities and functions are controlled or at least influenced by the brain, it is not surprising that its swelling disrupts many organ systems and activities, including special functions such as judgment, perception, and other complex mental activities. These are sensitive to even a little swelling, which (we hypothesize) may begin when oxygen supply is only slightly decreased because brain cells use more oxygen than most other cells. Mental confusion and hallucinations are very characteristic of severe HACE and are thought to be due to patches of edema in specific areas. Similar hallucinations occur in patients who have small strokes or small tumors in the temporal lobes, perhaps through a similar mechanism.

It also seems likely, since the stomach and intestines aren't obviously affected by oxygen lack, that the nausea and vomiting of mountain sickness are caused by malfunction due to lack of oxygen in the medulla, or midbrain, the more primitive part of the brain where the centers that control breathing are located. We consider that disordered breathing, so common at altitude, is due to changes in the sensitivity of the respiratory center and to conflicting messages coming from the carotid bodies. We speculate that altitude insomnia is due to disturbed "sleep centers," and that the staggering walk is due to edema of

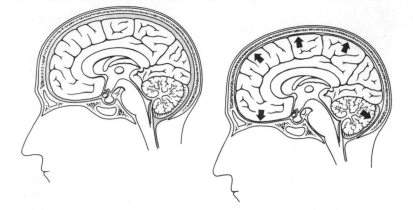

FIGURE 31. THE BRAIN IN ITS RIGID BOX

The soft whitish-gray brain is cushioned within the rigid hard skull by a thin layer of liquid — the cerebrospinal fluid — which is under pressure little greater than that of the atmosphere. Through the fluid are transmitted many of the chemical stimuli to and from the brain. The "markings" on the surface of the brain, defining its segments, are usually clear (*left*). When the brain swells (cerebral edema) because too much fluid is accumulating within the brain tissues, the brain becomes too big for its box (*right*) and presses against the walls, decreasing the brain markings and increasing spinal fluid pressure. But whether or not pressure is increased within the skull at altitude is still unclear.

cells that control posture. Quite possibly other disturbances, such as the increase in pulmonary artery pressure, may be partly due to malfunction of a nerve center.

If the brain swells within its tight case, it will compress the veins bringing blood from the eye through the small holes in the skull along with the optic nerves to each eyeball. By looking at the retina (the layer of light-sensitive cells in the back of the eye) at altitude, we will see that the blood vessels are distended with blood to twice their normal size, and often there will also be small hemorrhages. Brain swelling may be so great that the optic nerve head protrudes slightly into the back of the eye; we can see this bulging (called papilledema) with an ophthalmoscope, and it is a serious sign.

Physical examination of a patient with severe HACE may not be conclusive. The pupils of the eyes may be dilated and react sluggishly. The reflexes are usually normal but in deep coma may disappear. In other cases the victim becomes rigidly clutched in the fetal position (as was Bill), and occasionally he may have convulsions or violent spasms. In contrast to many infections of the brain, the neck is usually not stiff. Disorientation in time and place is often hard to detect, but sometimes it is spectacular. People who are able to control their emotions at sea level may behave abnormally when hypoxic, just as is the case with alcohol.

At 22,000 feet a very experienced climber aged fifty-four believed that he was by far the fittest member of the team and thus should go to the summit. In reality he was climbing slowly and clumsily; he was incoherent and at times quite irrational. When gently told he was not fit for a summit bid, he became very angry and soon had to be led down the mountain. His resentment lasted for years and he never realized how badly impaired he had been.

Hallucinations are dramatic evidence that something is very wrong. They are subjective — that is, perceived only by the patient, and thus may be concealed, denied, or blamed on fatigue or cold, or simply ignored.

A physician with considerable climbing experience wrote me a long letter describing hallucinations he had experienced while climbing at 14,000 feet. He heard voices talking to him and saw people walking nearby. He knew these were hallucinations and had sense enough to turn back, but even when safely down the sensations were still remarkably real to him. A few years later on another slightly higher peak, he had several days of much more severe hallucinations which he did not recognize as such; he became violent and had to be restrained. A tape recording shows how deranged he was, yet he denied this after returning home. A third episode, this time at 13,000 feet, though not as extreme, was also later denied.

Other climbers recognize their delusions at the time and recall them later as an interesting experience:

A strong young climber was soloing a moderately easy route at 12,500 feet when he felt, as he put it, "disembodied," as if he were watching himself from a distance. This other self thought, "I hope that fellow is being very careful." The climber could put this hallucination aside by concentrating on it, but when he turned his mind back to climbing, the hallucination again became real. He remembers this very clearly today.

Occasionally the hallucinations may be very vivid and graphically described. One famous climber offered candy to a person he believed was sitting near him; another talked quite rationally to an imagined companion. Other fancies are more farfetched:

The members who survived one particularly tragic climb said they had seen bulldozers and palm trees on the snow-capped summit, and that strangers were trying to steal their flashlights. Many days after the experience these bizarre hallucinations remained vivid and real.

Sometimes HACE comes on quite suddenly, despite what seems to have been a reasonably discreet rate of climb. The hallucinations may begin only after the victim is unconscious, but he may recall them later:

Twenty days after starting from 4,000 feet a small party camped at 20,000 feet, having "carried high and slept low" above their 16,500-foot base camp for ten days. One of the more experienced climbers (who had felt more tired and dizzier than the others for a day or two) fell asleep during supper, could not be roused next morning, and convulsed frequently for the next few days. He was eventually transported to a hospital where he recovered slowly, though some residual damage remained from blood clots. Years later he still recalls his hallucinations during the five days when he was unconscious and later remembered having had vivid hallucinations and a "stumbling walk" at 17,500 feet the previous year. On neither occasion did he have headache or cough or signs of pulmonary edema or in fact very much warning of impending trouble.

Did this expert young climber have a predisposition to HACE as some few do for HAPE? On both occasions he described, the rate of ascent and the climbing plan seem to have been safe, though he said later that the pace felt a bit fast for him. The "stumbling" was probably ataxia, an early warning sign. His hallucinations were particularly frightening and vivid.

Other parts of the brain may be affected, causing more obvious signs. In 1969 during the Mt. Logan studies, we noticed that some of the scientists coming down to Base Camp after a stay at 17,500 feet walked clumsily and staggered perceptibly, though they were otherwise quite well. At first we thought this was due to walking on loose gravel in Mickey Mouse boots (as the vapor barrier boots were affectionately called), just as on the mountain we blamed it on ploughing through deep snow, but soon we realized that it was an altitude effect that had not been previously described. Then a young Japanese climber was brought down after a much too rapid summit climb: he was unable to walk without falling, or to get his hands to do what he wanted them to do, or even to sit up, so impaired were his balance and coordination. For three days he lay in bed, too clumsy to feed himself, too unsteady to stand, though perfectly well otherwise; then he gradually recovered. Other climbers were beginning to realize that this clumsy walk was due not to boots or terrain but to something wrong with the brain.

Normally we are able to walk a straight line without staggering because a complex network carries signals from our feet, our eyes, and the balancing system (semicircular canals of the inner ear) to a part of the brain (cerebellum) where the signals are instantly sorted out and messages sent to muscles correcting any tendency to sway or fall. Hypoxia confuses the system, probably within the cerebellum. Today we recognize this staggering gait or ataxia as an early and important indication of hypoxia and attribute it to edema in or near the cerebellum. Impulses that coordinate arm, hand, and finger motion also pass to and from the cerebellum, and difficulty with these motions, as the Japanese climber showed, also occur, though less frequently; this is called dysmetria. A doctor wrote me:

I treated about 50 persons with moderate to severe AMS. They all showed improvement of sensorium with descent but I was struck by how persistent the ataxia was. It was striking to note complete lucidity, absence of nausea, and socially appropriate behavior coupled with complete inability to walk a step unaided. This often persisted for 12–24 hours.

Ataxia is easily tested for and is a good early warning of HACE. At altitude a person who cannot walk a straight line with heel against toe without staggering should be presumed to have early HACE. This staggering is quite different from the slow, clumsy, awkward motion so typical of the early stages of hypothermia.

Doctors working at the Himalayan Rescue Association Clinic at Pheriche on the route to Everest Base Camp have seen many cases of unconsciousness, coming on rapidly and with little other warning than staggering gait and mental confusion. Most who pass through Pheriche have headache, though it's not always severe. Almost invariably those individuals who have kept on, going higher and higher, usually too fast, without heeding the early warnings, are the ones who become victims, and some of them die.

A twenty-nine-year-old man flew to 9,000 feet and during the next week climbed to 14,000 feet, where he felt nauseated and lethargic but insisted on continuing. At 16,000 feet, nine days after starting his trip, he became unconscious and was evacuated with evidence of pulmonary edema and severe neurological signs. In the hospital he remained unconscious for ten days and still had evidence of brain damage six weeks later.

Such horror stories are uncommon, fortunately, but they would occur even more rarely if people appreciated how subtly altitude illness can begin. Hypoxia resembles overindulgence in alcohol: the person who has had to much to drink ("I'm perfectly all right to drive — just watch me") is like the mountaineer or skier who persists in going on despite impairment which should be obvious to those with him. On a mountain there may not always be a normal friend to take care of him, for almost everyone is affected to some degree. Mild cases of HACE are not unusual and certainly may improve spontaneously, but one can't ever be sure whether an individual will get better or rapidly worse. Any suspicious case should be treated as potentially serious.

Of course, it's important to remember that other causes of unconsciousness, headache, convulsions, or hallucinations can and do occur on mountains. Just because a person is at altitude does not mean his every symptom is due to hypoxia:

A healthy twenty-five-year-old man took thirteen days to reach 16,000 feet on a South American peak. During the next four days, on the way to 17,500 feet, he developed abdominal pain, fatigue, vomiting, fever, and diarrhea. At 18,500 feet, he related, "I was still the strongest member of our group. There was no warning.... When I woke up nothing worked on me too well, I couldn't think well and I couldn't talk too well...." During the next two days he was helped down to 13,800 feet, where he waited for helicopter evacuation for a few days, during which his temperature went very high. He lost consciousness during the flight and remained in the hospital for several months, regaining use of his arms and legs only slowly. Two years later he still had trouble talking, writing, and walking. His severe neurological problems are permanent, and it seems likely they were caused more by infection than by HACE.

A stroke (caused by bleeding or by clotting in the brain) or an infection like meningitis or encephalitis can act very much like HACE and can strike even a strong, active climber, sometimes affecting locals who might be expected to be better acclimatized than visitors. But altitude should be considered the probable culprit in any case of unconsciousness or brain malfunction unless or until proven otherwise.

As with HAPE, once HACE is suspected, getting down is the best treatment and in early cases improvement begins very soon; often the victim can go up again. More severe cases take much longer to recover and sometimes the damage is permanent. Oxygen promptly relieves headache — which returns just as promptly when oxygen is stopped. Ataxia isn't helped by oxygen and may last for several days after getting down — just why we are not sure since some other symptoms of HACE improve rapidly. Hallucinations disappear quickly, but the memory of them remains unusually vivid and the patient half-ashamedly admits to sometimes thinking them reality. Diamox may help, as it does in HAPE, but so far there's not enough evidence to prove this; in a tough situation it is certainly worth trying. It was used for a patient who had been comatose for a long time due to hypoxia from an anesthesia accident; the patient woke within minutes of receiving Diamox intravenously.

Dexamethasone, an adrenal steroid hormone, has been used because it was thought to improve brain edema caused by injury, but since it takes many hours to be effective, it's difficult to know whether or not it has helped, and it's no longer in vogue for trauma to the head. Brain edema from injury sometimes improves after solutions containing high-molecular-weight substances are given by vein, but they have not been used enough in HACE to make a judgment.

Some patients who have died from HACE have been autopsied. The brain tended to bulge through the incision, obviously swollen and heavy with fluid. There were many small hemorrhages on the surface as well as deep inside the brain. Such hemorrhages or clots are common after death from any cause and it is hard to know whether they occurred before or after death and how much they may have contributed to the illness.

Carbon monoxide kills because hemoglobin binds that gas 200 times as strongly as it holds oxygen, and thus it causes rapid, severe lack of oxygen, much like going very rapidly to high altitude. Headache is severe; mental confusion, clumsiness, and coma follow. At autopsy the brain is filled with fluid as it is in fatal cases of HACE. (The lungs often show edema too.) A few cases of deep coma from carbon monoxide poisoning have cleared quickly when hypertonic saline (a solution of 10 percent salt in water) was given by vein, but I know of no cases of HACE that have responded so well.

It seems repetitious but perhaps necessary to say that the best way to avoid HACE is to go up slowly, allowing the body time to adjust. People differ from one another — and the same person may be affected differently at different times. The speed of climb should be slow enough so that no one is badly affected. If one member of the party shows signs of HAPE or HACE, slow down, stop, or turn back before the problem escalates. There will be other days, other mountains.

The gratifying decrease in serious altitude illnesses in the Everest region (and indeed in most parts of the world) has come because people are learning about their bodies and their reactions to altitude. Alas, the increase in speed climbing or alpine-style ascents to very high summits is increasing mortality due to altitude, as G—— wrote:

Moving at this altitude (26,300 feet) was like wading through treacle. I became aware of a peculiar feeling of dissociation ... punctuated by ... momentary blackouts. A vicious headache gripped me.... I blacked out for twenty minutes ... woke momentarily and recall seeing P——. [They started down and he began to improve. Then P—— became ill:] Speaking in a slow whisper he told me he suddenly couldn't breathe.... His lips were very blue.... We had to get down and fast but a snail's pace was the best we could manage. [They somehow went on for several hours supporting each other as their strength ebbed.] About 10 P.M. P—— slumped and whispered that he could no longer see ... he had got too weak to walk ... he was so disoriented.... We slid down the last slope to camp.... P—— died a few hours later.

They had been moving for twenty-two hours. Both were excellent and experienced mountaineers. P—— was a doctor particularly interested and knowledgeable in altitude illness. They had climbed from 16,300 to 26,800 feet in two and a half days, then both had developed HACE, and P—— had HAPE as well. It was a predictable and avoidable tragedy. Sadly, there have been other cases like this among the best and boldest climbers. Those who dare to climb too high too fast must concentrate their all on the effort, oblivious to the beauty around them. They are courting death and disaster; one wonders whether the added thrill is worth the risk.

Chapter Twelve

OTHER ALTITUDE PROBLEMS

NOT EVERY ILLNESS on a mountain is caused by altitude — but a good many are or may be and these need to be sorted out. One that distends and distresses the climber is caused by decreased pressure (and dietary indiscretion). It is due to a law formulated by Robert Boyle some centuries ago and not yet repealed: the volume of a gas varies inversely to its pressure. Although doubtless recognized (though not appreciated) for many years, it has recently been dignified by a name: high-altitude flatus expulsion, or HAFE. The patient is less a victim than are his companions because the gas expelled is noisome. It would be unseemly (however appropriate) to call this "Boyle's disease."

Gas trapped anywhere in the body obeys Boyle's law, and ear or sinus pain sometimes follows aircraft flights; a tiny bubble in a recently filled or abscessed tooth can expand agonizingly during flight. Nitrogen will leave fatty tissue (where it is dissolved) and form bubbles in any part of the body if decompression is fast enough, causing "bends" or aeroembolism. But except for the possibility that tiny bubbles play some role in HAPE, trapped gas is more uncomfortable than dangerous on a mountain — at least so we believe today. The major problems at altitude are due to lack of oxygen rather than decreased pressure.

One of our body's natural responses to hypoxia is to produce more hemoglobin and red cells to transport more oxygen: soon after reaching altitude all the blood-forming organs go into high gear. The response is brisk and continues for weeks as an important part of the acclimatization process, usually turning itself off when the red cell count reaches 6 or 7 million cells per cubic milliliter of blood, up from the normal of 4.5 to 5 million. Another way of stating this is by the percentage of whole blood occupied by red cells — the hematocrit. The normal hematocrit is 40 to 45 percent; at altitude it may rise much higher and the blood may become thick and move sluggishly, the red cells stacking together like dishes, making their absorptive area smaller and thus decreasing oxygen transport rather than increasing it.

For this reason some mountain physiologists have suggested blood-letting (phlebotomy) when the hematocrit rises above 60 percent; on the few occasions this has been done the results were unimpressive. Robert Winslow and colleagues described a careful study of one native living at 14,000 feet in the Andes: enough blood was withdrawn (and replaced by an appropriate solution) to lower his hematocrit from 62 percent to 42 percent. There was considerable improvement in many functions, which led Winslow to suggest that even in highland natives, the optimal hematocrit may be as low as sea level normal, but there were so many interrelated variables that this important study needs to be repeated on more subjects. Several less careful studies on high peaks have given results that are equivocal at best.

Just the opposite approach was recommended some time ago: persons planning a high climb had a pint of their blood drawn and stored, and this was given back to them weeks later when high on the mountain. Here again nothing was proven, and there are certain risks in the procedure. Some have suggested that such "autotransfusion" might be good preparation for intense competitive sports, but it has been defined as "doping" and usually excluded by sports committees.

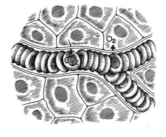

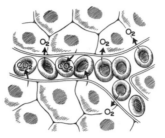

FIGURE 32. TOO MANY RED BLOOD CELLS
MAY BE DISADVANTAGEOUS

Until recently, the increase in hemoglobin and red blood cells which re-sults from long exposure to altitude has been considered a beneficial adap-tation on the grounds that more hemoglobin would carry more oxygen to tissues. Although Jourdannet found most high-altitude residents to be slightly anemic, Viault later found just the opposite. Most observers today feel that Jourdannet's subjects had other problems that made them anemic, for subsequent studies have found long-term altitude residents and accli-matized visitors usually have more than the normal hemoglobin.

But when the number of red cells increases considerably — as often it does — blood becomes thicker, moves more sluggishly, and tends to clot more easily in the small blood vessels. Thrombophlebitis (clots in veins) is a significant problem for persons with far too many red cells. In addition, the disc-shaped cells tend to lie flat against one another, decreasing their diffusing surface and thereby actually decreasing the oxygen available to tissues, as shown in the top figure. Whether or not withdrawing or diluting this thick, sluggish blood is helpful at great altitude is still debated, but we are coming to believe that too much blood may be an adverse adaptation and perhaps no better than too little.

The very complicated machinery that causes (and prevents) blood clotting is affected by hypoxia and by the dehydration so common on high mountains. Blood platelets (important in clotting) are probably increased during hypoxia (although a few studies have found them decreased), while other studies show that fibrinogen (another major factor in clot formation) may be either increased or decreased. Not only is the blood thicker, not only does it move more sluggishly, it also tends to clot more rapidly and easily. The first I ever heard of this came in a personal experience many years ago:

We had been climbing for weeks and were within striking distance of the summit of K-2 when a severe storm pinned us in our tents at 25,000 feet for ten days. We were unable to melt snow and had little water or food and became weak and very dehydrated. One of the stronger climbers developed a blood clot in one leg, then in the other, and soon bits had broken off and been carried to his lungs. He was lost in a fall during our desperate attempt to carry him down.

Immobilization in his sleeping bag, dehydration, a high hematocrit, and increased coagulability stimulated by hypoxia caused his blood clots and the resulting tragedy. Many similar cases have been reported since then. Quite often while a victim of HACE or HAPE is being laboriously transported to the hospital from some high mountain, he must lie immobile on a stretcher for long hours; clots form and may determine the outcome:

A strong climber who developed HACE at 20,000 feet could not be evacuated immediately, and during a long carry-out developed clots in his legs which migrated to both lungs. A week later, when he reached the hospital, he was seriously ill because of these clots, though his HACE had cleared. Years later he still has problems with the obstructed veins in both legs.

Clots can form even in active climbers and sometimes they are hard to recognize and may masquerade as HACE:

The day after carrying a load (using oxygen) high on Everest, a vigorous doctor who had been to 25,500 feet the year before woke unable to see to the right and with weakness in his right arm. At no time did he have headache. During descent his right leg became paralyzed for a time, but when he reached base camp forty-eight hours later he was almost well. Several days later he had severe vertigo, double vision, vomiting, and weakness. He was evacuated by helicopter and recovered partially, but for several months had some neurological abnormalities. He returned a year later to 20,000 feet without any problems.

This man may have had a small hemorrhage in his brain that sealed off spontaneously, or, more likely, he developed small clots that in time were bypassed by the opening up of new blood vessels. Whatever happened may have been aggravated by drinking too little fluid so that his already thick blood became even thicker and more likely to clot. It's difficult even in the best circumstances to tell the difference between a blood clot in the brain and a hemorrhage, so in his case, as in most others on a mountain, the exact explanation eludes us. Quite a few persons (native Sherpas as well as Europeans) have had this kind of stroke at high altitude and some have died.

It is hard to reconcile this tendency to clot with the reports so common in the last century of bleeding from the nose, eyes, and ears and even through the skin during alpine climbs; perhaps the difference in altitude or extent of dehydration is responsible. Perhaps whether one bleeds or clots at altitude depends on which of the adversary substances discussed in the chapter on HAPE predominates.

In 1968 one of the members of the Mt. Logan High Altitude Physiology Study became unconscious soon after climbing to the 17,500-foot laboratory. He was airlifted to a hospital where he rapidly recovered. One unexplained observation was the presence of a number of small hemorrhages in the retina of each eye. I was unsure of what this meant, but a few weeks later one of the scientists complained of spots before his eyes and I saw hemorrhages there too.

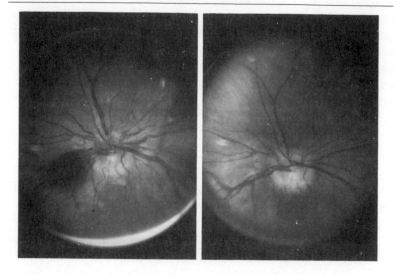

*FIGURE 33. THE RETINA AND ITS BLOOD VESSELS
AT SEA LEVEL AND AT ALTITUDE*

Using a strobe light flashed through the lens of a special camera, photographs can be taken of the retina of the eye, which appears as above right. The round light-colored area to which the small arteries and veins (*dark lines*) lead is the optic disc, or head of the optic nerve, which carries light and color impulses from the sensitive retinal cells to the brain.

Above 15,000–16,000 feet the veins and arteries almost double in diameter, and blood flow in them also doubles (*above left*). This appears to be a universal and "normal" response to altitude (and in fact to hypoxia from other causes as well). In addition, over half of all people going above 17,000 feet have small hemorrhages in various layers of the retina (*above left*) due to leakage or to actual rupture of small vessels. Some are quite large and blob-shaped; others are small and flame-shaped. Though alarming at sea level, these hemorrhages at altitude rarely cause symptoms and usually disappear within a few weeks, leaving no residual damage.

This led to detailed studies over the next ten years. We soon realized that many, perhaps most, people going to 17,500 feet would have hemorrhages in their retinas, but these usually caused no symptoms and disappeared within a few weeks.

Since then hemorrhages have been found in many mountaineers on many expeditions. They are rare below 14,000 feet but become more and more common the higher one goes. We wonder what they mean: if the eye is window to the mind, are there hemorrhages in the brain too? If so, are they important?

One possibility is that they might be caused by tiny clumps of platelets that have lodged in a small vessel in the retina, obstructing it and causing a "blow-out." Perhaps the increased flow and pressure in retinal capillaries stimulates discharge of substances, some of which increase while others decrease platelet clumping and change the "tone" and leakiness of the capillary, much like what happens to cause capillaries of the lung to leak in HAPE. Is it reasonable to assume (although so far without experimental observations) that this process which we are confident happens in the lung may also happen in the brain, eyes, and other parts of the body? These questions are among many that cry out for answers.

Mosso described periodic breathing at altitude and correctly attributed it to lack of oxygen. Physicians saw it in debilitated patients and called it Cheyne-Stokes breathing; some thought it a predictor of imminent death. We know today that the periodic breathing at altitude, and a similar pattern in the dying patient, are caused by a kind of schizophrenia in the control of breathing.

In the brain is a collection of specialized cells called the respiratory center, which is very sensitive to too much or too little carbon dioxide and responds by increasing or decreasing breathing. But one of the major sensors for oxygen is located elsewhere — in the neck. If you feel gently below the angle of your jaw, closer to the front than to the back, you can feel your pulse as blood is pumped through the large carotid arteries to the brain. At one place along the artery there are two tiny sensors which detect changes in the passing blood and generate important signals. One of these sensors (the carotid sinus) reads changes in blood pressure and is one of many "baroreceptors" in the walls of arteries throughout the body. If the blood pressure rises, these sensitive receptors tell the brain to signal the vessels to relax, lowering the pressure; if pressure falls, they signal the blood vessels to constrict. The carotid sinus, located so close to the heart, is ideally situated to detect changes in the blood pressure as soon as they begin. Pressing on the carotid sinus will slow or even stop the heart, but it is probably not affected by hypoxia.

Another nearby sensor-regulator — the carotid body — may be more important at altitude. There's one on each side of the neck, each weighing less than an ounce, each made of specialized tissue called glomus cells densely packed with mitochondria. The fact that each receives about thirty times the blood flow that goes either to heart or brain suggests that they may be quite important. Their blood comes directly from the carotid artery and is but a heartbeat away from the heart and lungs. The carotid bodies are thought to read the oxygen level in the blood, and when it falls, to increase both rate and depth of breathing. Normally the carotid bodies and the respiratory center in the brain work harmoniously to maintain normal oxygen and carbon dioxide levels, but they may also oppose each other. For example, as oxygen falls, the carotid bodies dictate increased breathing. This lowers carbon dioxide, which leads the respiratory centers to call for a decrease in breathing. But if oxygen falls too low, the carotid bodies apparently have override power. Maintaining oxygen has a higher priority than maintaining normal carbon dioxide.

The carotid bodies seem ideally placed to monitor oxygen since they receive blood immediately after it leaves the lung, in comparison to the respiratory center, which is a second or two farther away. It seems logical to have the sensor that can take corrective action when oxygen falls as close as possible to the lungs, while the less critical response (to changes in carbon dioxide) is a bit more distant. There are other sensors, and obviously this description is oversimplified.

The hypoxic ventilatory response, or HVR for short, is a descriptive term used to identify the strength with which an individual's ventilation controls react to a decrease in oxygen. The HVR varies between individuals and in the same individual under different circumstances. The HVR tells us how a person will breathe if oxygen in the blood falls below a certain threshold. If the HVR is brisk or strong, breathing will be increased, whereas if the HVR is blunted or sluggish, breathing isn't changed and the impact of oxygen lack is greater. But that threshold may be lowered (blunted) by fatigue, starvation, certain drugs, and perhaps by a long stay at altitude. How sensitive the HVR is to lack of oxygen is important in determining how well or poorly the individual reacts to lack of oxygen at the time, but because it is affected by many things, it is not a completely reliable predictor of who will and who will not get sick.

Are the carotid bodies the site of the hypoxic ventilatory response? Do people with a brisk HVR have larger than normal carotid bodies? Is the opposite also true? Do people who can't adjust to altitude have small or poorly functioning carotid bodies? These important questions can't be answered completely today. We do know, however, that large carotid bodies are found in some races of high-altitude natives, but whether similar enlargement occurs in long-term visitors is unknown. Interestingly, there are no data indicating that the respiratory centers in the brain change during long exposure to altitude or to sea level hypoxia.

The HVR is blunted in some people born to generations of altitude residents and in at least some sojourners who stay for weeks or months at altitude. Such blunting may be the basis of an unusual form of altitude illness — chronic mountain sickness, sometimes called Monge's disease after the man who first described it sixty years ago, Carlos Monge, Sr. It is an uncommon problem that occurs after months or years of residence at altitude. Here is one of the cases Monge described:

A forty-eight-year-old native resident at 14,000 feet complained of increasing shortness of breath for three years. She became unable to

*sleep except sitting up and developed swelling of her feet. She was
weak and had vague pains in her chest. When examined, her skin and
lips were a dark dusky red color, she had signs of fluid in her lungs,
and a red cell count of 7.5 million compared to 6.0–6.5 million, which
is average at this altitude. She remained in the hospital at altitude and
died a month later.*

A similar picture may be seen, but the cause may be different, as in the following case:

*A fifty-one-year-old miner who had lived all his life at 14,000 feet
developed fatigue, weakness, shortness of breath, occasional swelling
of his feet, and vague pains in various parts of his body. His skin and
lips were dark purplish red, his red cell count and hematocrit were very
high, and the right side of his heart was enlarged. He had several unconscious spells and occasional hallucinations before he went to live at
sea level, where he slowly improved.*

A quite different problem can cause a similar medical picture at sea level:

*A forty-three-year-old truck driver lost his job after falling asleep at
the wheel several times. He was overweight, had a dusky red color to
his lips and skin, and was sluggish and drowsy all the time. His blood
count and hematocrit were high and his heart enlarged. While being
studied he died suddenly during sleep.*

Carlos Monge, Sr., considered the first patient typical of the affliction that has since borne his name. The second patient is not quite so typical and part of his problem was likely due to emphysema from his exposure to mining dust. The third patient had "sleep apnea syndrome," a recently identified problem which in a milder form probably affects more people than we now realize. All three had disturbed breathing patterns because their responses to lack of oxygen and/or accumulating carbon dioxide were abnormal, probably because their hypoxic ventilatory responses were blunted. Many persons with sleep apnea are fat and inactive; they are constantly drowsy and fall asleep at inconvenient times. These features led to the name "Pickwickian syndrome" after Dickens's character, but now that we know more about them we use less picturesque names.

Accumulating data indicate that many, even most, cases of chronic mountain sickness are due to weak ventilatory drives, perhaps blunted by long residence at altitude. As a result the victims breathe less and have lower oxygen levels in the alveoli and blood and thus are effectively living at a considerably higher altitude. We say they suffer from alveolar hypoventilation. Their carbon dioxide levels are higher, but the carbon dioxide drive (which is usually strong) may be blunted too, with the result that they simply don't move enough air. In an attempt to compensate, the number of red cells increases, blood becomes thicker and more viscous (and harder to pump), and blood clots are common. Pulmonary artery pressure is higher than usual for that altitude, and over time the pressure backs up into the heart, which enlarges and eventually fails.

What is particularly fascinating about alveolar hypoventilation — whether we call it that or Pickwickian syndrome or Monge's disease — is that it occurs at sea level too as a common affliction that can be devastating, as the third case shows. One form is called sleep apnea, but another, more common, is known as intermittent upper airway obstruction, or IUAO, which is a fancy name for snoring, though some causes of IUAO are due to obstruction elsewhere in the upper respiratory tract. The unfortunate snorer, whose snorts and roars may be legendary, spends part of each night with less oxygen in his blood as he struggles for many seconds to take a breath. In effect he may go to altitude for part of each night. No wonder he is sleepy during the day! Pulmonary artery pressure increases during each period of hypoxia and over the years may become permanently high; the heart enlarges and fails, and we have a condition that is hard to tell from Monge's disease.

Many studies have shown that periodic breathing at altitude can be eliminated almost completely by taking Diamox at bedtime: this "smooths out" the irregular breathing, sustains arterial oxygen at a steady level, and gives more restful sleep (except for the few who get a strong diuretic effect from Diamox). Does Diamox work as well for the snorer? Almost certainly not, alas. For Monge's disease? We don't have enough information.

With more and more people spending more and more time at altitude, new problems are surfacing — though one is not really new at all.

A twenty-nine-year-old man climbed Mt. Rainier (14,400 feet) in two days, experiencing only a mild headache. At 5,000 feet on the way down he had a series of "blackouts" (loss of vision but not loss of consciousness) lasting about thirty seconds and coming every ten minutes. He blamed them on the hot day and after an hour or two he recovered completely. A year later, taking seven days to reach 14,500 feet on Mt. McKinley, he had the same experience. He was given Diamox and continued the climb to the summit. Taking Diamox on subsequent climbs, he has had no further trouble.

This frightening episode was blamed at the time on lack of oxygen and improved after several minutes of breathing supplementary oxygen. Another case suggested a new wrinkle to an ancient affliction:

During his youth a forty-five-year-old engineer (who understands some physiology because his doctoral research had been in arterial blood flow) had repeated attacks of flickering vision (called scintillating scotomata). Doctors said he had a form of migraine. After fifteen to twenty years without attacks they began again, accompanied by inability to talk clearly and often by complete blindness. This happened several times a month, usually on a mountain. After an especially bad attack when he could not talk or move or see while on a difficult rock climb, he was thoroughly examined and no abnormality was found. Though he had no headaches, the neurologist said he was having migraine equivalents, not related to altitude.

I now know of a dozen episodes like this. Because they seemed to occur on mountains, they were blamed on oxygen lack. A search of the medical literature on migraine turned up reports of hundreds of patients with similar blind spells or scintillating scotomata with and without headache, occurring at sea level and therefore not due to oxygen lack. Although historical reports of migraine go back at least to biblical times, its exact mechanism is still not fully understood. We are confident that a massive change in blood flow to the brain occurs, but why or in which direction and at what stage in the attack is debated. Perhaps on a mountain the change in cerebral blood flow due to hypoxia triggers these migraine equivalents, but should we classify them as "altitude illness" when they occur at sea level as well?

It happens that just before and during a classic migraine attack platelets tend to clump together, though we don't know what sets this off. Since aspirin prevents platelet clumping, it might possibly relieve a migraine attack. It does not affect classic migraine, but the equivalents seem to be different.

Because of aspirin's anticlumping action, the second patient was advised to take one aspirin a day for prevention. He did so for three years, resumed climbing, and had no attacks — until he grew careless, forgot the aspirin, and immediately began having attacks. Now, again taking one aspirin a day, he has no more migraine equivalents and has been climbing frequently for several years.

The best we can say of such evidence is that it is suggestive and interesting; much more information is needed.

Some unusual forms of hemoglobin have already been discussed, and the illnesses they may cause can be not only serious but also hard to diagnose:

A forty-five-year-old black social worker learned she had sickle-cell disease after the birth of her third child when her anemia was slow to improve. After the fourth child she had several "sickle-cell crises" during which she had pains in legs and abdomen. She attended a meeting at 9,000 feet and developed severe abdominal pain, which she suspected was a sickle-cell crisis, but because she lived at 5,000 feet, it took some time to persuade the doctor who took care of her that alti-

tude was responsible for this crisis. With descent and appropriate care she recovered. Similar milder attacks have occurred when she has tried to go to altitude since then, though she flies in commercial aircraft without trouble.

This intelligent woman is fortunate in knowing her problem and being able to interpret the signs and symptoms accurately. Others are not so fortunate:

A young white mechanic took a long bus trip from sea level to 7,000 feet and within two hours of arrival developed nausea and severe pain in the left upper abdomen. During the next three days he grew worse, and after special studies showed that his spleen was abnormal, it was removed and a diagnosis of sickle-cell disease was proven. Given oxygen he recovered slowly and returned to sea level.

This young man's father drove from sea level on hearing of his son's illness and within three hours developed somewhat similar symptoms, was given special tests and also had his spleen removed, and the diagnosis of sickle-cell disease was confirmed. He too improved with oxygen and descent. Only at this point was it learned that "according to the patient, miscegenation in his progenitors was likely."

Sickling has very rarely been reported in a person without some black or Mediterranean ancestry, though the relationship may be quite far back. If signs and symptoms at altitude are not typical and suggest sickle-cell disease, remember that unlikely diagnoses may be necessary if common ones can't explain the problem.

An eighteen-year-old man went from sea level to 5,500 feet and a day later developed pain in his abdomen, which grew worse in the next five days. He was hospitalized and after special studies was found to have sickle-cell trait, which improved when he returned home, only to strike again when he went back to 5,400 feet. He came from Dutch and Sicilian ancestry.

Another white male flew to Denver from sea level and in a few hours noticed abdominal pain. He went to 7,000 feet for a brief visit and on return to 5,400 feet, after some jogging, noticed that the pain was worse and he was hospitalized. Again special tests showed sickle-cell trait and he returned to Florida, where he has since been well. Both his father and a paternal uncle have had similar episodes. The family are of Belgian, Spanish, and Italian descent.

These and the four similar cases reported recently by Peter Lane and John Githens are genetically of white stock with no evidence of black ancestry, showing that nonblack persons may have the sickle trait and suggesting that they may be more susceptible to serious problems when going to altitude.

Some mountain tragedies are impossible to classify, though they are more likely than not a bizarre form of altitude illness:

A young woman had diarrhea and vomiting after a ten-day walk to 15,500 feet. She became very weak and was carried on a yak down to 14,000 feet, where she seemed to improve, taking plenty of fluids and a soft diet. But when she resumed the descent she became weak and had to be carried. During the night she became irritable, withdrawn, irrational, and soon unresponsive. She was carried down to 10,600 feet and given oxygen, but slipped into coma and died.

If this poor woman died of HAPE or HACE it took an unusual form and course. But what she did have cannot be explained from the information available.

A twenty-one-year-old trekker had flown to 9,000 feet and taken a week to reach 14,000 feet, though he had difficulty keeping up with his group. There he treated his diarrhea with large doses of Lomotil and a tranquilizer and became lethargic and unsteady on his feet. Next morning he could not be roused. He was given oxygen while evacuation was being arranged and twenty hours later woke up. Though irrational for a short time, he improved and later walked down unaided.

This patient probably was developing HACE and aggravated his problem by taking too much strong medication. Most medicines are more powerful at altitude (alcohol among them), and doses should be adjusted carefully. There are several stories of climbers who have taken sleeping tablets and wakened during the night confused or irrational, left the tent, and fallen to their deaths. Tranquilizers and sleeping tablets should be avoided — or only a small dose taken.

Quite frequently other factors complicate response to altitude — dehydration or medication in the preceding case reports, but others as well:

A young medical student went to the Andes to work in a small community clinic. After a few days at sea level he was flown to 12,000 feet. He complained of nausea, headache, diarrhea, and fatigue, but his host blamed this on food and after a few days drove him up to his clinic at 14,000 feet. He felt worse, seemed confused and went to his small room, lighted the space heater because of cold, and went to bed. Next morning he was found dead, the gas heater was out, and autopsy showed he had died of pulmonary edema and carbon monoxide poisoning. He probably died from HACE and HAPE as well as carbon monoxide poisoning.

A number of near tragedies have been caused by exposure to carbon monoxide at altitude, due to poor combustion of fuel used in a cooking stove in a tightly closed, nearly impermeable mountain tent. It's important to remember that carbon monoxide will replace oxygen in combination with hemoglobin and can cause severe or fatal hypoxia. Even smoking, by preempting oxygen with carbon monoxide, contributes to lack of oxygen at altitude.

Confronted with more and more unusual stories about illness or death at altitude — almost any altitude — we should attribute them to the effects of oxygen lack unless or until proven otherwise. But they should be investigated:

A young woman was said to have developed what certainly sounded like HAPE after climbing Mt. Washington (6,400 feet)! I was skeptical, knowing no other proven case at such a low altitude. The hospital would not release her record and she would not answer my letters. I learned later that she had a heart condition — perhaps damage to the mitral valve, which, together with the strenuous climb, might have caused pulmonary edema — if she had anything at all.

Is our increasingly mobile society exposed to risk by flying in commercial aircraft? This is an interesting but difficult question. Jet aircraft fly from 25,000 to 45,000 feet, depending on the duration and direction of flight and where the jet stream happens to be flowing. But the cabin pressure is maintained at a pressure equivalent to between 4,500 and 7,000 feet, rarely as high as 7,500 feet. This altitude isn't risky for those who get around reasonably well at sea level, but it's quite possible for someone like the father and son mentioned above to develop a sickle-cell crisis on a long flight. Some of the children with an absent pulmonary artery, who may develop HAPE at 5,000 to 6,000 feet, might also be at risk during a very long flight, such as from New York to Tokyo, where one may spend seventeen hours at altitude. All commercial flights have oxygen available, and it would be prudent for these unusual individuals to ask in advance to have oxygen nearby — or even to bring their own equipment, as some of those who are severely hypoxic at sea level are accustomed to doing.

This raises more wide-ranging questions: Who should not go high? Can we accurately identify those more likely to be badly affected? Many persons who in years past would never have considered or been able to take a trip to the mountains have been patched up and can lead quite active lives. Wheelchair patients are no longer uncommon in mountain resorts. How should their doctors advise those who wonder about going to the mountains?

Those most at risk are patients with heart or lung problems. In general, persons who are moderately active — and with few symptoms at sea level — can tolerate a visit to 8,000 to 10,000 feet, taking the same precautions urged on the healthy. Some people with high blood pressure may need to adjust their medication, those with well-controlled heart disease need to be a little more careful about exertion. The multitude with asthma, emphysema, chronic bronchitis, and other lung problems do quite well at moderate altitude, sometimes even feeling better in the cleaner air than at sea level, providing they can lead reasonably active lives at home. Those who are more handicapped won't do so well and probably should not go high.

Special problems need special consideration by the individual's doctor — who we hope will be knowledgeable about altitude too! It's safer and easier for doctors to be conservative and advise against a mountain visit, but they should know that many persons with a variety of problems are surprisingly well at altitude, and the enjoyment from such a visit may outweigh any small risk. Age alone is no barrier. Some believe that young children are more susceptible. At the other extreme, the very old may have problems because arteriosclerosis reduces blood flow (and oxygen) to the brain: the added hypoxia of altitude may aggravate their problems.

Conception and pregnancy have some special features at altitude. Apart from the possibility of miscarriage or premature delivery, which can happen anywhere, anytime, there's no added hazard at moderate altitude for the mother. The problems begin at 14,000 feet and some people believe even as low as 10,000 feet. They can be summarized as follows:

· Fertility is decreased in long-term altitude residents but returns to normal if the woman returns to low altitude. Sperm counts and motility tend to be slightly decreased in men living at altitude.
· Prematurity is increased, and birth weights are lower in children born at altitude if the mother has been there for all or most of her term. Though most studies have shown that children born of altitude natives also tend to have lower than normal birth weights, one recent study shows the reverse!
· Some minor birth defects are reported by some observers to be more common in childen conceived and born at altitude, and mortality before and after birth is higher.
· Children born at altitude, or taken there in early life, may be slightly better acclimatized than those born at sea level and taken later to altitude.

What should her doctor tell the newly pregnant woman about altitude? Already she is warned about smoking, alcohol, coffee, most medicines, and so many environmental dangers that her life seems an endless list of prohibitions! Should we add altitude to this list? Not surprisingly, there are different opinions. When we remember that the fetus at sea level is living in an oxygen environment roughly equivalent to that on top of Everest, it seems unlikely that going from sea level to 10,000 feet will make much difference. But some careful observers feel that even this adds slightly to the risk for the fetus. Above 10,000 feet fetal oxygen will be further reduced, and it seems prudent to counsel the pregnant woman not to go higher than that.

Though conception is slightly less likely at altitude, there are few specifics. The Spaniards were said to be infertile for fifty years after the conquest of Peru — but closer reading suggests that they produced pregnancies that miscarried or babies who died at birth. One possible world record I have been unable to verify:

While stormbound at 25,000 feet in the Himalayas, a famous woman climber is said to have become pregnant by her French tentmate. When I asked someone who knew them, he answered, "I don't know, but a Frenchman is capable of this."

Since birth control pills are known to increase the risk of blood clots, fertile women should probably discontinue contraceptive pills several weeks before a mountain expedition. This increases the possibility of pregnancy and a woman may ask about the danger to a fetus conceived at altitude, but unfortunately we do not know.

What constraints should be placed on persons with illnesses other than those that may interfere with oxygenation? Special circumstances such as recovery from surgery or a heart attack must be evaluated individually by the doctors most involved. Roughly the same principles apply: if one can get about reasonably well at sea level, moderate altitude is no real problem.

Above 10,000 feet the rules change. People marginally active lower down should probably not venture so high. The higher one plans to go, the more careful a doctor must be with advice. I get many calls from those who desperately want to climb a Mexican volcano or an Andean peak, going to 18,000 or 20,000 feet, usually on an easy route. Some have been forbidden this pleasure because of a minor heart murmur, a prolapsed mitral valve (very common but usually unimportant), diabetes, epilepsy, arthritis, and on and on. It's not wise to generalize about these; only careful study of the individual can give a reliable decision.

The fact remains that most people who get along at sea level will benefit from being in the mountains — if they don't go too high or too fast and if they listen to what their bodies are telling them. Those who wish to enjoy the mountains should learn how to stay well while there, how to detect early warnings of altitude sickness, what to do about them. Those who wish to go much higher, climbing among the greatest splendors of the world, are a different breed: they must learn much more, they must be more thoughtful of themselves and others, and they must weigh risks against benefits most carefully.

Chapter Thirteen

ACCLIMATIZATION

ARE THE MEN AND WOMEN who have stood on top of Everest breathing only the high thin air about them different from the rest of us? Do they have some secret ingredient in blood or tissue, or do they react differently to lack of oxygen? What if anything do they share with the thousands who are equally short of oxygen from illness at sea level? Or with the millions who are born, live, and die three miles high in the Andes or Tibet?

Alexander the Great and Cyrus and his chronicler Xenophon crossed high passes and fought or traded with the natives, but they made few references to mountain sickness or to the capabilities of the natives. Perhaps they were preoccupied with more pressing matters, like freezing or starving to death or fighting. Marco Polo mentioned the stamina of high-altitude ponies, but he didn't relate this to the thin air that made his campfires burn weakly. Acosta painted a graphic picture of mountain sickness, and since he traveled extensively in the high Andes for several years, he probably noticed that those who stayed at altitude for long did not have these symptoms. Yet his only reference to acclimatization is dependent on the translation: he seems to have said that those who ascended from the east (which took a long time) fared better than those who came up the quick steep route from the west, and he may have been the first to appreciate that slow ascent might enable the body to adjust to altitude. Humahhad Haidar in 1550 was more specific: altitude residents did not suffer from *dam-giri* (the Tibetan name for mountain sickness).

Acclimatization, according to the encyclopedia, refers to gradual adjustments made to any alien environment — hot or cold, wet or dry, high or low — and means a series of changes in a living organism that enables survival in conditions otherwise lethal. It's a gradual process, taking weeks or months or perhaps years; some believe it is perfected only after generations, and that only those who acclimatize survive and bear progeny — be they plants, animals, or man. Human acclimatization to altitude is no different: it takes time and it is also quite an individual process. Some persons adjust easily and well, but others take longer, while some never really get used to altitude. The unfortunates who develop Monge's disease probably represent failed acclimatization.

The immediate reactions to abrupt oxygen lack are "struggle responses" by which the body tries to keep the oxygen flow to cells as close to normal as possible. They include increased breathing, faster heartbeat, increased number of red blood cells, opening of capillaries, and more subtle changes. These are the sorts of responses that Claude Bernard had in mind when he emphasized the importance of the "constancy of the internal environment" and showed how we depend on such emergency reactions to maintain our physiological status quo. Struggle responses suffice for a few hours or days, depending on the altitude, while the slower, more sustainable changes are maturing. Alexander von Muralt called these struggle responses "accommodations," while Alberto Hurtado preferred to speak of "natural" or "acquired" acclimatization as he saw it in altitude natives and visitors respectively. Today we use the term *acclimatization* for changes which develop in weeks or months, and reserve *adaptation* for those which take generations.

The distinction between acclimatization and adaptation was

the subject of a rather heated exchange that took place about fifty years ago (and continues more moderately today). In 1925, after working for many weeks at 14,000 feet in Peru, Joseph Barcroft (who knew as much about high altitude as any Englishman at the time) wrote:

> *The acclimatized man is not the man who has attained to bodily and mental powers as great in Cerro de Pasco as he would have in Cambridge (whether that town be situated in Massachusetts or England). Such a man does not exist. All dwellers at altitude are persons of impaired physical and mental powers.*

Carlos Monge, Sr., was outraged. Not having access to the paper he published in Spanish at the time, I can only imagine what he told Barcroft then, but years later he was still angry and wrote:

> *For our part, as early as 1928 we proved . . . that Professor Barcroft was himself suffering from a sub-acute case of mountain sickness without realizing it. His substantial error is easy to explain as resulting from an improper generalization on his part of what he himself felt and applying his reaction to Andean man in general. . . . Andean man must be physically distinct from sea level man requiring much further research before one may define, let alone apply, the terms inferior and superior.*

Acclimatization was confused with rapid adjustment or accommodation by two famous explorers, Robert and Adolphe Schlagintweit, who traveled far and high in the Himalayas surveying for the government of India in the middle of the nineteenth century, and wrote:

> *. . . so far as the symptoms to be considered in acclimatization, we can speak from our personal experience. When we crossed passes at an elevation of 17,500 to 18,000 feet for the first time we felt serious symptoms. A few days after, when we had traversed the highest points and passed several nights at these altitudes, we were almost completely free of these disagreeable symptoms, even at the elevation of 19,000 feet.*

Though these famous travelers had been in the mountains for some time, "a few days" is too short a time for real acclimatization, and they were more likely adjusted or accommodated.

During this same period Denis Jourdannet (Paul Bert's friend) spent twenty years studying the people and country of Mexico and found those living in the highlands to be anemic (though elsewhere in his book *The Anemia of Altitudes* he contradicts this). Noticing the stocky build of these highlanders, he described "the vast chest [which] makes him comfortable in the midst of this thin air ... ," an observation echoed almost a century later by Barcroft in the Andes. Jourdannet's writings caused quite a storm among entrepreneurs who were contemplating establishment of a French empire on the high plateaus of Mexico, and a French military surgeon, Dr. L. Coindet, was sent to investigate. He wrote that the natives had the same respiratory and pulse rates as the more recently arrived French, but acknowledged that the natives could do more strenuous work and for longer. Bert drew on Jourdannet and Coindet (and many others) when he predicted that an increase in red corpuscles (which he showed carried oxygen) and an increase in breathing (in volume per minute if not in rate) would be important to acclimatization.

Here is beginning recognition that natives born at altitude are different in some ways from sea level natives sojourning at altitude because they have adapted (in the Darwinian sense) by changing over many generations. The descendants of altitude natives are thoroughly at home up to 17,000 feet (the highest permanently inhabited villages) and can do hard physical work even higher, as Barcroft wrote after visiting a mine over 250 feet deep:

Every few minutes like a bee out of some hive in cold weather, someone would appear from the mouth of the mine. He would be much out of breath, he would take frequent pauses on the way up, but the weight on his back would be a hundred pounds ... he would sit for a while to rest and then down into the mine again he would go to bring up another load.

The first major medical expedition to a high mountain came about almost by chance, as Yandell Henderson, a young professor from Yale, wrote after attending an international physiology meeting in Vienna in 1910:

For me the greatest event was to meet Haldane and Douglas whom previously I had known only from their papers. All one afternoon and evening we discussed respiration, and it was during that talk that Haldane told me of his wish to spend sufficient time on some high mountain to study the development of acclimatization. . . . "I want a nice comfortable, easily accessible very high mountain with a fairly good hotel on top" said Haldane. And I replied "Come to America next summer and we will spend a month or two on Pike's Peak."

And so began the first of many studies on 14,000-foot Pikes Peak. Edward Schneider joined Haldane, Douglas, and Henderson for a month on the summit, where they measured respiration and alveolar gases at rest and during and after exercise and charted Cheyne-Stokes breathing. Above all they talked about pulmonary and circulatory physiology for endless hours. Young Henderson, entranced in the presence of these giants, wrote much later:

To those of us who were privileged to participate in the Pike's Peak expedition the memory of that time has remained a life-long inspiration. . . . It was a golden time. Men who are friends under 460 mm of barometric pressure are friends until the end of life.

These four men shaped generations of students and scholars, and their happy communion was possibly the most lasting heritage of that summer. Haldane still clung to his belief that a major component of acclimatization was the ability of the lungs to actively secrete oxygen, so that blood leaving the lungs would actually contain more oxygen than was in the alveolar air. Haldane persisted in this belief even after Barcroft analyzed his own arterial blood and alveolar air during eight days in a "glass house," in which the percentage of oxygen in the air was gradually reduced to simulate ascent to 17,000 feet. Haldane argued that Barcroft was not fully acclimatized.

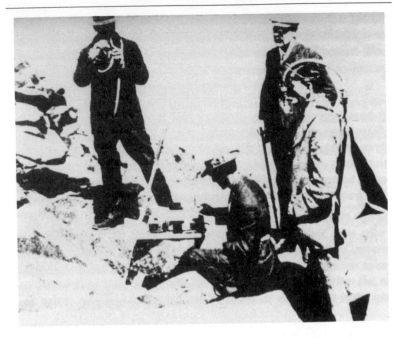

FIGURE 34. HALDANE AND FRIENDS ON PIKES PEAK IN 1911

Although de Saussure, Mosso, and a few others had made some short-term studies of human reactions on high mountains, the expedition to Pikes Peak inspired by Yandell Henderson was the first to examine changes during many weeks of residence at 14,000 feet. Members of the expedition are shown here collecting, in large rubber Douglas bags, the air exhaled during a period of exertion on top of Pikes Peak. They also collected samples of alveolar air for analysis by catching the last portion of the deepest possible exhalation. The clinical observations of each other and of the hordes of tourists arriving by train, mule, or on foot are particularly interesting when compared with what we see today. A remarkable young lady, Miss Mabel Fitzgerald, accompanied them to Denver, but it was not thought fitting for her to remain on the summit unchaperoned. Instead she traveled through the mining camps of Colorado, and a few years later through the Great Smoky Mountains, carrying her equipment in saddlebags on her horse; she collected and analyzed alveolar air samples from hundreds of long-term residents at altitude, a profile of data that has never been duplicated. Many other mountain expeditions have tried to match the standards set by this early and splendid effort.

To refute this, Barcroft went off to Peru with seven equally distinguished physiologists to spend several months in the Andes, and brought back proof that arterial blood contained less oxygen than the alveolar air in newcomers, residents, and natives. The number of subjects was small, and his technique might be criticized because the alveolar air and arterial blood samples were not taken at the same time, but nevertheless this was the final blow to the secretion theory — which seems sad: it is rather an attractive concept! Barcroft recognized the importance of increased breathing: it washed out carbon dioxide, making more space for oxygen in the lungs. He calculated how much oxygen was transported at different levels of saturation and increasing numbers of red cells. And he introduced the intriguing concept of "mean capillary oxygen pressure" — an idealized number which, if it prevailed throughout the body, would represent the oxygenation of the whole body. Barcroft's book *Lessons from High Altitude* is charming and scholarly, as is Henderson's *Adventures in Respiration*.

The next major study of acclimatization was done in 1935 on the Peruvian Andes by a large international expedition led by Bruce Dill. The party concentrated on the physico-chemical changes of blood in natives and in acclimatizing sojourners. Many of the papers that came directly from this splendid expedition are landmarks in our understanding of the chemical changes that permit man to live at altitude.

World War II halted mountain research but energized scores of studies of acute hypoxia because aircraft could go higher than their crews, whose lives depended on oxygen when flying at altitudes that gave the most tactical advantage. Even a momentary interruption of the oxygen supply meant unconsciousness or death. Aircrew had to be trained to fear hypoxia and to detect its earliest subtle touches. Before this training was adequate many pilots perished — some unaware that their night vision was reduced to half that at sea level when they were flying at 10,000 to 12,000 feet, others because they failed to realize what was happening. Some were too confident: "I've been to 20,000 feet many times and it never bothered me a bit" was one refrain not only from older pilots who had flown for years, but also from the young and overconfident.

Our task as teachers was to show them realistically what lack of oxygen could do, and we did this by setting up in the decompression chamber a model airplane with a stick and rudder like their actual aircraft controls. The pilot was asked to "fly" this little model after he had removed his oxygen mask at 25,000 feet but to replace the mask immediately if he noticed anything at all wrong with his "flying." In my unit, which ran perhaps 55,000 pilots and gunners through this program, we asked one or two men from each group to do this demonstration, and I can't recall more than a dozen out of 2,500–3,000 who were able to put their mask back on before they fell unconscious, even when we ordered them to do so. Using a real machine gun mount, we did a similar demonstration for turret and waist gunners. They too got religion fast!

But this was very acute hypoxia, not a hazard one is likely to encounter in peacetime life. Flight commanders soon asked whether any medicine or exercise could protect aircrew, giving them not only greater tolerance for accidental loss of oxygen, but also more tolerance above 45,000 feet, where even breathing pure oxygen was not enough because the barometric pressure was so low. This would not be acclimatization as we use the word today, but accommodation or adjustment. We tried taking pilots up in the decompression chamber once or several times a day, each day a little higher without oxygen, hoping they could develop adjustments that would carry over — but it didn't work: they only became more tired. Soon that effort became moot with the advent of pressurized masks, and later with pressurized cabins. Interestingly, this tactic has been revived by Soviets and Japanese seeking to preacclimatize for high Himalayan climbs.

At war's end it would have been unfortunate if all the energy invested in altitude research were dissipated, and it was not. Many of those who would later contribute mightily to what we know about oxygen and man were blooded in these military aviation training and research programs. As for me, my interests were in climbing rather than flying, and I was able to seduce the U.S. Navy into a study that was more relevant to mountaineers than to aviators; this is the subject of chapter 15. Others went back to their clinics and laboratories. Mountaineering was about to enter a new era.

In 1950 the country of Nepal, closed to foreigners for centuries, opened most of its highest mountain ranges to climbers, and what we might call the Golden Age of Himalayan climbing began. The new generation would go on to feats we could not conceive. Medical research did not lag far behind.

Griffith Pugh, a prominent British physiologist, led a small party to Cho Oyu in 1952 primarily to gain experience with oxygen equipment for the attempt on Everest, which he accompanied the following year. Pugh and others brought back a wealth of data from these two expeditions, some from as high as 25,000 feet, enabling Pugh to predict that on the summit of Everest without extra oxygen a man would be able to do very little physical work: staying alive would be difficult enough no matter how well acclimatized he might be. Two decades later this prediction was confirmed when the first men reached Everest's top breathing only air. Even though they were breathing supplemental oxygen, the first summiters, Hillary and Tenzing, were weak and near exhaustion on the summit.

Pugh was back in the Himalayas in 1961 as scientific leader of an extraordinary expedition which included some of the finest British and American mountaineers and physiologists. A prefabricated insulated hut was erected at 19,000 feet not many miles from Everest and continuously occupied for five and a half months. Some of the party stayed as long as nine weeks without descending, though others had to go down to 15,000 feet to rest and recuperate. Despite good food and comfortable living conditions, all of the party lost weight, and they concluded that 19,000 feet was too high for long-term living — a conclusion shared by some altitude natives! Their studies

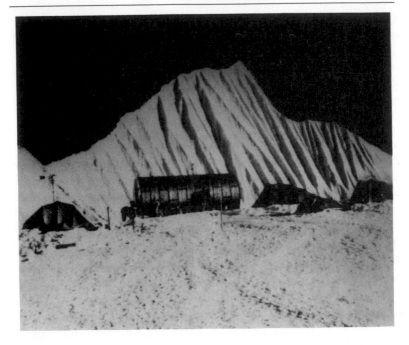

FIGURE 35. THE SILVER HUT—NEAR EVEREST IN 1961

In the winter and spring of 1960–61, British and American mountaineer-scientists occupied this spectacular site at 19,000 feet near a shoulder of Ama Dablam, one of the beautiful peaks south of Everest. During the four months, they examined many of the changes in themselves caused by exposure to high altitude. In the "Silver Hut" they were protected against the cold and wind and could do a number of sophisticated studies on heart and lungs and blood, at rest and during work. They had good food and were able to get ample outdoor exercise skiing and climbing nearby, but nevertheless they all lost a great deal of weight, strength, and ambition, and concluded that 19,000 feet was too high for long-term acclimatization. From this study came a great deal of insight into the physiological changes which occur at great heights. There are no permanently inhabited villages above 17,000 feet.

confirmed what had been found on Everest and Cho Oyu, and added much more:

After weeks at altitude lack of oxygen was still driving respiration despite the lowered blood carbon dioxide, but the respiratory center had become more sensitive to carbon dioxide — as it is at sea level. . . . Newcomers were as physically fit or even fitter after a few weeks at altitude as those who had been there for months. . . . Physical work seemed to be limited by fatigue of working and respiratory muscles and the heart could only work at about two thirds its sea level capacity. Diffusion of oxygen from lung to blood was also a limiting factor at 19,000 feet.

Pugh's party also managed to do two maximum exercise tests at 24,400 feet, thus putting two more points on the curve predicting work capacity that had been drawn up by Pugh on Everest and by Rahn and Otis earlier.

These observations were dramatically highlighted just a year later when Chinese armies crossed their troubled border with India high in the northwestern Himalayas; maneuvers and skirmishes occurred at altitudes as high as 12,000 to 16,000 feet in very difficult conditions. The Chinese had been living on the high Tibetan plateau for many months or years and were acclimatized to 15,000 feet; the Indians, on the other hand, were hastily moved to altitude by truck or aircraft from the low Indian plains. The result was predictable: it is said that the Indians suffered more casualties from altitude illness than from enemy action. On the asset side, General Inder Singh and other Indian doctors soon published the most extensive collection of cases of altitude illness yet reported. A few years later, Singh wrote a paper on acclimatization that has become a milestone in our progress to understanding. Sujoy Roy, an Indian cardiologist, published a small book of respiratory and circulatory measurements made on highland natives and new arrivals.

Military men around the world must have been startled by what happened on that high faraway frontier, and one hopes that they learned never to attempt military action by unacclimatized troops taken too rapidly to altitude. This had not been a problem for mountain troops in the two world wars or even in the Korean engagement, but since the Indian experience the American army has been actively involved in high-altitude research, particularly on Pikes Peak; other groups too have worked there and on White Mountain (California), Mt. McKinley (Alaska), and elsewhere. Altitude physiology is flourishing.

From 1967 to 1979 the Arctic Institute of North America, supported by grants from the National Institutes of Health, carried on research in a summer laboratory at 17,500 feet on the snow plateau near the summit of Mt. Logan in Canada. At first we were interested in trying to define exactly what caused mountain sickness and how it could be prevented. But the laboratory was supplied by air, and the shock of flying from 2,000 to 17,500 feet in less than an hour made almost everyone too sick to make this protocol safe. After a few years, and some rather frightening episodes, we turned to acclimatization instead, studying subjects who had climbed the mountain slowly and then spent several weeks at Logan High. From this research came the first reports of high-altitude retinal hemorrhage. The value of Diamox for smoothing out periodic breathing during sleep was confirmed, and forty papers defining various aspects of life at altitude resulted. One of the more valuable long-range benefits was the interest in altitude research inspired in more than a hundred young people who participated.

During the sixties and seventies Himalayan climbing increased furiously; speed climbing at dangerous altitudes became popular, and hordes of unsuspecting tourists could be — and were — flown too rapidly to dangerous altitudes. Hundreds became sick and many died — not only tourists but experienced mountaineers as well. John Dickinson and Peter Hackett organized the Himalayan Rescue Association, which established a small clinic at Pheriche several days' march

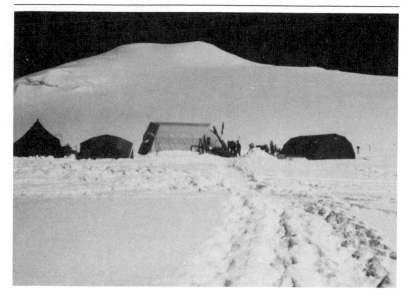

FIGURE 36. "LOGAN HIGH"—THE ARCTIC INSTITUTE'S ALTITUDE LABORATORY

From 1967 to 1979, the Arctic Institute of North America sponsored a summer program on Mt. Logan, Canada's highest peak. At first the goals of the study, which was supported by the National Institutes of Health, were to examine some of the biochemical changes in altitude illness. But it very quickly became apparent that flying to 17,500 feet from near sea level was much too dangerous, so the whole study was changed to look at the processes of acclimatization. The first laboratory was used for several years before it sank deep into the thousand feet of snow which fill the summit bowl on Mt. Logan. Thereafter a new set of buildings had to be erected every year.

---

below Everest Base Camp. There volunteer doctors from several countries took care of the sick and collected a great deal of information about altitude sickness. Even more important, their teaching program impressed many people with the risks of altitude and undoubtedly prevented much illness and many needless deaths. They and others have taught trekkers and climbers about the serious pathology that can develop at altitude — and how to avoid it.

A large and elaborate Italian expedition to Everest in 1973 not only managed to get seven men to the summit but also made extensive studies of work capacity and metabolism in thirty-six men during a long stay at 17,500 feet. Even more ambitious was the American Medical Research Expedition to Everest, the first party whose primary motivation was science rather than reaching the summit, although two members of the party did so. A well-equipped and comfortable laboratory was set up at 17,500 feet and another one at 20,700, where most of the exercise studies were done. Blood was drawn on several climbers at higher camps and brought down for analysis; Chris Pizzo obtained alveolar gas samples from himself on the summit, breathing air (though he had used oxygen during the ascent). The party studied what factors controlled breathing at altitude in the acclimatizing Europeans and in the altitude natives (the Sherpas) while awake and asleep. The capacity for work at altitude was measured, and hormone, intestinal absorption, and psychometric studies were also done. But few actual measurements were made at the highest altitudes, and the extrapolated predictions have been challenged by some.

In 1982 Bill Mills obtained a generous grant from the state of Alaska to establish a combined rescue clinic and research laboratory at 14,000 feet on Mt. McKinley. This great mountain attracts increasing crowds of mountaineers (from an average of fifteen climbers a year in 1950–60 to 800 each year recently), and many were being hurt or killed — and dozens required treatment for altitude illness. Hackett, Mills, and others set up the High Latitude Laboratory to treat altitude illness, frostbite, hypothermia, and injuries, and to serve as a base from which rescues and evacuations could be mounted. It became an ideal site for research in altitude illness, but had no advantage over Pikes Peak for studying acclimatization.

The McKinley laboratory is well supplied by aircraft and the scientists have accomplished a good deal, but even there it is difficult to transport and use certain sophisticated instruments to obtain critically important data very high on a mountain. The climbing scientists are always at the mercy of weather, transport, cold, and many other obstacles that interfere with experiments and data collection at extreme heights. Though mountain laboratories are the "real world," where people live and work and sleep and are exposed to many stresses, it has slowly became clear that one cannot tell whether some of the adverse effects attributed to altitude might be due at least in part to cold, dehydration, exhaustion, inadequate food, and a host of other unpleasant influences. It was time to study hypoxia in its pure form, in a more sheltered laboratory setting. The decompression chamber, bigger of course than the small cylinders used by Paul Bert for altitude studies, would be ideal. Such studies had been done in 1946, and were repeated in 1985; they are described in chapter 15.

Disregarding the impact of cold and other mountain stresses, what exactly happens to a mountaineer as he goes from sea level to the highest point on earth? Let's assume that the party flies to 5,000 feet and from there takes three weeks to reach 18,000 feet and climbs more slowly in stages from there to the summit.

The long up-and-down approach march will toughen his muscles, strip excess fat, and gradually accustom him to slightly less oxygen every few days. As he passes 10,000 to 12,000 feet he will be aware of increased breathing, pounding pulse, and usually a headache (indicating that his brain is getting more blood than at sea level in an effort to compensate for the lowered oxygen). The fortunate also notice increased urination (recognized a century ago by German physiologists and called *hohendiuresen*), a favorable indication that the kidney is putting out more water and sodium bicarbonate (an essential step in acclimatization), while those with weaker struggle responses may go on to develop one of the forms of altitude illness discussed earlier. If the climber continues slowly, allowing time for acclimatization to develop, his bounding pulse lessens, breathing is a bit easier, the headache goes away, and he feels better and can do more.

These changes are due to adjustments in the oxygen transport system that are triggered automatically somewhere around 7,500 feet by a decrease in oxygen in the thinner air.

The first and most important contribution comes from increased breathing stimulated by lowered oxygen in blood sensed either by the carotid bodies or by the respiratory center in the midbrain or both. Deeper and/or faster breathing brings more air deeper into the lungs, washing out carbon dioxide and making more room for oxygen. Up to a point, the more air the climber moves, the greater will be the oxygen pressure deep in the lungs — but if the carbon dioxide falls too low, unpleasant dizziness, numbness and tingling, faintness, and even unconsciousness will follow. This is a rather common occurrence in excitable people who hyperventilate at sea level. At altitude the lowering of carbon dioxide by natural overbreathing is compensated by excretion of bicarbonate in urine.

The effect of increased breathing on the oxygen cascade is to decrease the oxygen pressure drop or gradient between outside air and that deep in the lung, bringing alveolar oxygen pressure closer to that at sea level. This is the first and most important response in acclimatization.

Oxygen must now cross the barrier between alveolus and blood in the lung, and at this stage the pressure drop — the Alveolar-arterial (A-a) gradient — is normally quite small. There's little change in most people during acclimatization, at least until around 25,000 feet, but some individuals, perhaps more than we now appreciate, accumulate fluid in the wall between alveolus and blood even at low altitude, slowing oxygen diffusion and increasing the A-a gradient. We call this interstitial edema, and it may occur in everyone but be so minor that it is not noticeable. We measure the A-a gradient by drawing arterial blood and simultaneously sampling alveolar air, which is not exactly the kind of thing one does every day on a major expedition or during a vacation dedicated to recreation, and so it is not a practical way to detect early interstitial edema. The bottom line is that the A-a oxygen gradient is usually small and plays only a small part in acclimatization — though it may be pivotal at extreme altitude near the summit.

In the next stage — carriage to the tissues — oxygen easily enters the blood and combines loosely with hemoglobin, leaving only a small amount in physical solution. Little or no oxygen is lost in this process or during passage from large to smaller and smaller arteries and finally into the capillaries, barely big enough for the red blood cells to tumble through in single file. The oxygen cascade is not affected. But four important factors besides oxygen pressure affect how much oxygen reaches the cells: these are essential components of both adjustment and acclimatization.

The first of these is the amount of hemoglobin in the blood. Hypoxia stimulates formation of a hormone called erythropoietin, which in turn stimulates formation of hemoglobin and red cells in bone marrow, so that more hemoglobin and red cells are formed as altitude increases. It's fascinating to find that production of erythropoietin is "turned off," and only replacement red cells are made, when the number reaches a level that presumably the body finds optimal. If erythropoietin is not turned off, then further increase in red cells is counterproductive and a bad adjustment. Perhaps even a moderate increase in red cells is not as favorable as we have previously thought. But when everything runs smoothly, enough more carriers become available and more oxygen can be carried by a unit of blood.

Next, the speed with which these carriers move changes. Immediately on arrival at altitude the rate and force of the heart increase, thus increasing the volume of blood per stroke per minute — the cardiac output. This remains high for a few days or a week and then falls to or below normal as other accommodations develop.

The third factor is a substance called 2, 3, DPG, which lies on the surface of red blood cells and increases the avidity with which they attract oxygen. DPG is increased during hypoxia and may play a part in improving the carriage of oxygen, though there's some debate about how important it is.

Finally, the Bohr effect mentioned in chapter 6 becomes important in both lungs and tissues. Simply stated, as carbon dioxide leaves the blood in the lungs, hemoglobin attracts more oxygen, and as carbon dioxide diffuses from cells into blood in the tissues, oxygen leaves hemoglobin more rapidly. The Bohr effect shifts the oxy-hemoglobin dissociation curve to the left in the lungs and to the right in the tissues and is a neat added touch in transport and delivery of oxygen.

The argument over the position of the dissociation curve has been going on for years. A rightward shift enables hemoglobin to pick up oxygen more readily, and to release it more rapidly when oxygen pressure is somewhat lower than normal. The leftward shift has little effect on pickup, but allows hemoglobin to hold oxygen more tightly until its pressure (in the capillary) is very low, when a large amount of oxygen is rapidly released. Currently available data make it difficult to decide which shift is better at altitude because most of the studies have been done under quite different conditions. Robert Winslow examined the shape of the curve on acclimatized climbers during the American Medical Research Expedition to Everest and concluded that well-acclimatized persons could maintain the curve close to its normal position. Hebbel found many years ago that persons born with a mutant hemoglobin that gave them a lifelong leftward shift seemed to tolerate moderate altitude better than normals. Perhaps it's significant too that the bar-headed goose, which flies easily to 30,000 feet, and the llama and alpaca, which live at 14,000 to 16,000 feet, like many other mammals native to high altitude, all have left-shifted hemoglobin dissociation curves compared to their sea level relatives. The argument may be moot: it seems likely that a right-shifted curve is beneficial up to moderate altitudes (12,000 to 14,000 feet), while above this a leftward-shifted curve is better.

There are different kinds of hemoglobin (page 100), and some animals native to altitude, like the yak, have two types of hemoglobin, one "fast" and one "slow" in acquisition of oxygen. Just how helpful this is in acclimatizing the yak to altitude is unknown. The deer mouse can switch from a high-altitude form of hemoglobin to a low-altitude form depending on whether he is in Death Valley or on a high peak where he may go for the summer. Substances are now available that change human S-hemoglobin to the fetal type, and it seems likely that something of this sort might someday help patients irreversibly hypoxic with disease.

The final stage in the oxygen transport system is passage of oxygen from the tiny capillaries into cells. Capillary walls in the tissues as in the lung are thin and offer little resistance, but they are separated from cells by an interstitium or loose network containing fluid through which oxygen must diffuse. The greater the distance through the interstitium, the greater the drop in oxygen pressure. Obviously there's an advantage to having capillaries closer to cells, and an early "struggle response" when one goes to altitude is the opening up of inactive capillaries. During acclimatization new capillaries are built so that all cells will be closer to their oxygen supply.

Once inside the cell, oxygen is avidly used by the mitochondria, the little factories where every life function is energized, and the more of them there are, the more each cell can produce. There is some evidence that another step in acclimatization may be an increase in the number of mitochondria, at least in some animals, but much more work must be done before this is certain. If there were an increase in the number of mitochondria, it would not affect the oxygen cascade at all, but it would enable more oxygen to be used, thus increasing extraction of oxygen from blood before it returns to the lungs. This does happen in acclimatization.

In addition to a steady supply of oxygen, tissues need assurance that when a sudden call comes for a large increase, it will be available. Ordinarily, as we start to exercise and the muscles require more oxygen, the heart rate speeds up and more blood is pumped to meet this demand. An additional supply of oxygen is available in the muscles, loosely bound to myoglobin. During acclimatization, myoglobin increases substantially, and we might think of this as a storehouse or a facilitator of oxygen transfer, even though each molecule of myoglobin (like hemoglobin) holds less oxygen than at sea level. It's interesting that myoglobin has a very left-shifted oxy-hemoglobin dissociation curve, admirably suited for release of a lot of oxygen rapidly when the local supply gets very low.

These are the major changes in oxygen acquisition, transport, and delivery that tend to bring the oxygen supply to the tissues closer to that available in the air. We can summarize them in a table that applies to the sea level resident arriving at moderate altitude and staying a few weeks:

Major Changes in Acclimatization

Increased breathing	Better exchange of air in alveoli
Increased cardiac output (temporary)	More blood is moved
Decreased cardiac output (later)	Enables more oxygen to be acquired (especially during work)
Increased red cells	More carriers available for oxygen
Increased tissue capillaries	Blood is brought closer to cells
More mitochondria in cells	More units swing into operation
Enzyme changes	Oxygen is used more efficiently
Increased myoglobin	More oxygen is locally available

There are many other more exotic changes within each cell, in specialized tissues like the glands, which produce hormones, in the kidney, which discards bicarbonate as an important contribution to acclimatization, and in the heart. These don't seem to have as much impact in bringing tissue oxygen closer to that in the outside air as the major changes we have looked at.

Slow gradual ascent, "packing high and sleeping low," is the traditional mountaineer's way to acclimatize best. It gives the body enough stress to push the responses, but not so much as to precipitate mountain sickness. It is time-tested and it works for most people, but not for everyone. For reasons we don't fully understand, some people don't do well above 20,000 feet; they never regain their well-being, and their work capacity never reaches that of their companions. We suspect this is due to a blunted respiratory drive: the victims do not respond to low oxygen with the greater breathing others do. Undoubtedly there are more causes for such flawed acclimatization, but they elude us today.

In recent years the slow "siege" tactics of establishing a series of camps higher and higher while acclimatizing have become less popular than alpine-style rushes, where one or two persons acclimatize by making shorter day trips from base camp, climbing from perhaps 18,000 to 22,000 feet or higher, returning each night. After a few weeks they may have gained enough acclimatization to make a dash for the summit.

This is very different from "going up" in a decompression chamber for a few hours a day and returning to sea level at night, a tactic used by Japanese and Soviet climbers who claim that it helps, but have little hard data to prove it. American and Canadian physiologist-mountaineers believe that the altitude where you sleep is more important than where you spend the day. This is just as true in acclimatization as it is in determining whether or not you will get mountain sickness. "Pack high and sleep low" applies only if you sleep just a few thousand feet lower; it is not the same as returning to sea level after a few hours at simulated altitude in a decompression chamber.

Alpine style requires stamina, skill, and daring; it is not for everyone. Only those who are fit and very strong, who can move up and get down fast enough before altitude sickness can catch them should try it. In addition to HAPE and HACE, alpine-style climbers face exhaustion, dehydration, and hypothermia, all of which reinforce the effects of hypoxia. The wave of the future seems to be to climb in small, cohesive parties, taking time to acclimatize and enjoying the greatest mountains with less risk. Few mountaineers would like to eliminate the spice of danger, or turn away from stretching of limits, but death from altitude illness seems a foolish way to go.

Folk wisdom among old Himalayan hands has it that each trip to altitude becomes easier, that the body "remembers" how to acclimatize and does so more rapidly and completely on each expedition. This is not unreasonable when one thinks of all the other acts or functions we "remember": how to ride a bicycle or to play the piano, or incidents associated with a smell or a sound; we "remember" to sweat when afraid, to blush at certain memories, and so on. Why should we not remember how to acclimatize?

In addition to the mountaineer, others must go from sea level to altitude to work or to fight or to live at 10,000 to 14,000 feet for months or years. The acclimatization process is the same; over time the changes mature more completely, but along the same paths. But the sea level native never reaches at altitude the full capability he had at sea level, nor does he match the native born at altitude.

How does this person, born of generations of altitude natives, differ from the well-acclimatized sojourner? It is interesting that different races seem to have followed slightly different paths over the centuries, but for most the basic responses are the same, though some may be slightly muted. All involve the same oxygen transport system but emphasize different sections.

Start with the fetus: it is totally dependent on its mother's blood, from which oxygen must pass through the placenta to the fetal circulation. We can calculate that fetal oxygen supply is equivalent to what a person would breathe at 30,000 feet! The fetus has two major advantages that help adjustment during nine months' residence in such an hypoxic state. The most important is elimination of the gradient of breathing since oxygen is received directly into arterial blood. Another is the more efficient transport of oxygen because the fetus has hemoglobin that is sharply left-shifted and delivers oxygen in bulk for a small tissue pressure drop. We can only speculate about other processes, but clearly the fetus is an expert in acclimatization.

Suppose the mother is acclimatized to 17,000 feet — a true native: what of the fetus? Lorna Moore thinks that the fetus conceived and carried to term at altitude is further acclimatized, as evidenced by its birth weight, which is higher than that of the fetus delivered by a short-term visitor to altitude. But the high-altitude newborn, however long its mother has been acclimatized, weighs less, and the mother is more likely to have complications during her pregnancy, than at sea level.

When we look at long-term, Darwinian adaptation we find variations between different races, some of them well recognized, others still unclear or controversial. There's hard evidence that some animals develop larger alveoli if born at altitude. Less firm evidence suggests that this may be true of humans born of generations of altitude residents. These adaptations improve oxygen uptake by providing more area for diffusion and are more effective than simply developing a larger chest capable of moving more air in and out, an adaptation favored by Andean natives but not by Tibetans.

Sherpas (descendants of generations of altitude residents) seem to have a less sensitive response to oxygen lack (the HVR) than do sea level natives, but this has not been adequately studied nor do we know enough about other altitude natives to generalize. On the other hand, Andean natives have larger than normal carotid bodies, suggesting that they may respond more briskly to the hypoxic challenge.

Sherpas don't have more hemoglobin than their sea level cohorts, whereas Andean residents of the Quechua-speaking family do. Tibetans are more comparable to Andean natives, but we don't yet know enough about their hemoglobin to tell whether Tibetans may have a "fast" and a "slow" type — like their versatile servant, the yak. Sherpas whose forebears lived on the high Tibetan plateau now live at somewhat lower altitude; their oxy-hemoglobin dissociation curves are left-shifted, like the Himalayan bar-headed goose! Sherpas seem able to do more work at extreme altitude than can even well-acclimatized sea level natives, but there are few well-controlled studies to support this, and when the chips are down, willpower, motivation, spirit are probably more powerful spurs to summit Everest than is a slightly better level of acclimatization.

It seems to me that many exciting adventures in human physiology are waiting for students of the faraway peoples who have adjusted to altitude (or to cold or heat or drought) along different genetic pathways. From them I am sure many lessons can be learned that could affect all of us.

We must now look at some practical aspects of acclimatization: How long does it take? How long does it last? How can it be speeded up or enhanced? And, of special interest, is it helpful to acclimatize at altitude for competitions held at sea level? To compete at altitude, where should one train — and how? Only partial answers are available for such questions and individual variation makes a great deal of difference.

We can say quite confidently that for most people a month of gradual ascent is enough to acclimatize well to 18,000 feet. We can also say, though less confidently, that above 20,000 feet deterioration outstrips acclimatization and those who stay for months so high do not improve with time. (John West told me of an Andean caretaker who has lived at 19,500 feet for two years with three companions who have not been there quite so long: they go down to 13,000 feet to play football once a week!)

No other people are known to live for more than a few months above 17,000 feet, but perhaps harsh conditions contribute to their failure to thrive.

For the less adventuresome, taking only a few days for the ascent will protect against illness up to 10,000 feet, and in less than a week most people feel almost as they do at sea level. Full acclimatization of course takes longer — but ten days will see you well on the way.

There are not many firm data about how long it takes a person to lose acclimatization once acquired, but most of the changes — even the blood count — return to normal values within a week or two of returning to sea level. It is interesting that shortness of breath on exertion may last for a week or longer at sea level after altitude residence, because the alkaline reserve (base excess) has been depleted.

When we try to decide what is an optimal level of hemoglobin we are on uncertain ground. Crude efforts have been made to increase hemoglobin and improve altitude tolerance by transfusing blood into the acclimatizing mountaineer: the results have been conflicting. Others have tried removing what might be called excess hemoglobin and replacing the blood with plasma. Again no clear result. Sound theory and a lot of anecdotal evidence suggest that a hematocrit of less than 58 percent is optimal, but we can't conclude from this that removing blood is beneficial.

We can convert adult-type hemoglobin to the fetal or fast type, but this is still justifiable only in certain serious illnesses, and so far no method has been considered for the healthy mountaineer. Undoubtedly, tinkering with the ability of hemoglobin to pick up and release oxygen may help in some situations — but not today, not yet.

Though acetazolamide (Diamox) apparently improves altitude tolerance and decreases illness, we are not ready to call it an "artificial acclimatizer." Several expeditions have used Diamox every day, but their conclusions vary and the studies have been totally uncontrolled (in the medical sense!). From what I know today I suspect that taking Diamox regularly during a major climb may be more helpful than harmful — if one insists on taking some kind of medicine. There may be a risk: some of those who have taken Diamox regularly and stopped it abruptly while at altitude developed severe acute altitude problems rather unexpectedly.

Other medications that improve oxygen acquisition and transport have unpleasant side effects. Provera (a female sex hormone that stimulates breathing, especially during pregnancy) does improve oxygenation — but the resulting feminization is not appealing to all. Other respiratory stimulants have not been adequately tested.

Where should one train for competition at altitude? Can you improve sea level performance by training at altitude? Do altitude natives surpass sea level natives in competition at sea level? At altitude? Here there are few firm answers. So intense are competitive athletics today that even the smallest edge is important. One cannot train to the utmost limit at altitude as one can at sea level because even at 5,000 feet work capacity is less than at sea level. Acclimatization lowers alkaline reserve, thus giving carbon dioxide and lactic acid more influence on respiration: the well-acclimatized individual must ventilate more than his sea level rival from the same exertion. An advantage comes with a moderate increase in hemoglobin, which can deliver more oxygen per unit of blood pumped. But too much hemoglobin makes blood too sluggish.

We should be able to draw conclusions by comparing Olympic performances in 1968 at 7,300 feet in Mexico City with those in Los Angeles in 1984, but so far no one has been able to give a definitive answer as to where one should best have trained for those events. At Mexico City the largest number of records were broken in short, intense events (less than two minutes). Runners don't breathe at all during the hundred-yard dash, so altitude made little difference (unless the thinner air offered a trace less resistance). In most longer events, performance was below that in the Games held at sea level. But it's difficult to compare records set years apart because of the steady improvement in performance throughout the world of sports during the last twenty years.

One might find an answer by comparing Denver-based professional teams with those from lower altitude, on the assumption that if there were an advantage to training at altitude, the big money involved would so dictate. This has not happened. Our Olympic skiers trained at 5,000 feet, but no conclusions as to benefit have been forthcoming. For several years runners and prospective expedition mountaineers have trained while breathing low-oxygen mixtures for a few hours at sea level each day. This is roughly the same as spending time at simulated altitude in a decompression chamber, but in this country at least that tactic has not proven to be of value.

Though the answers to these important questions are not yet firm, we can draw a few conclusions that are today rather generally accepted:

· Beginning above 5,000 feet the maximum work one can do decreases by about 3 percent per 1,000 feet of altitude and improves only slightly during months of altitude residence. Endurance or submaximal work does improve slightly over time, but does not exceed the limit noted above.
· Training at altitude cannot be quite as intense as at sea level and the competitive edge thus may be slightly dulled. Training above 8,000 feet therefore is of little value.
· Advantage does come from increased hemoglobin (and its oxygen-carrying capacity) resulting from a stay at moderate altitude, but this is at least partially offset by the decrease in buffering power that comes with acclimatization and perhaps by the increased viscosity of blood.
· Athletes training for short, intense events do not benefit from training at altitude; those planning to compete in endurance events at altitude should train for weeks at that altitude.
· Some altitude natives do surpass their cohorts in sea level

competition, but others do not, and the explanation is more likely their lifelong dedication to running rather than their level of acclimatization.

· Intermittent hypoxia for a few hours a day does not produce acclimatization, and there is little evidence that it improves performance.

What, if any, relationship does altitude acclimatization have to the changes that make survival possible for persons severely hypoxic from chronic lung disease? What about those who have sleep apnea, or Pickwickian syndrome (alveolar hypoventilation), or who have lost a lung to disease or surgery? Or those who cannot breathe adequately due to polio or other muscular weakness? Are there some solid lessons from high altitude research that apply to these unfortunates? This is a complicated issue: in some conditions the defect is an increased barrier between alveolus and pulmonary capillary, increasing the oxygen gradient (and often causing retention of carbon dioxide too). In others the problem is inadequate lung capacity or weakness of respiratory muscles causing poor ventilation, or inadequate respiratory stimulus. I can't hope to cover these issues here; they are sophisticated medical problems beyond the horizon of this book. But I believe, and strongly, that much of what we find on mountains may be relevant to sea level.

Finally, what of the longtime altitude resident who returns to sea level? Will he have trouble deacclimatizing? The answer is firmly no — he easily adjusts in a few weeks. The mountaineer coming home from high in the Himalayas is euphoric and elated. Simple things like green grass, flowers, warmth, and space to move about delight him. Life is a precious, many-splendored thing, filled with joys and surprises. But within weeks the trivia of everyday intrude: there is money to deal with, the daily round is dull and uninspiring compared to the high drama of a strenuous climb where a single purpose dominates. Depression is common, divorces or broken liaisons are likely, life loses some savor. It has been tempting to blame this on lasting effects of hypoxia, but those returning from a fantastic voyage at sea or across vast deserts, or from any major trial, have experienced similar effects. They are more likely due to shifting gears.

Acclimatization to altitude is a wondrously complex process where many interlocking changes enable survival under extreme conditions. When we look at sea level man and observe how within seconds he becomes unconscious when deprived of oxygen, the wonder grows that he is able to get anywhere near the harsh and hostile summit of Everest. We wonder even more that whales can dive without breathing for an hour, that turtles can hibernate for months underwater, that the lungfish can go for years without breathing. The adjustments of such animals go far beyond us.

Equally remarkable is the "acclimatization" at sea level which enables patients with congenital heart disease or acquired lung disease to be quite active, even though their blood oxygen level may be as low as (sometimes even lower than) that of the mountaineer on the high Himalayas. Here is an area for study that is still largely unexplored.

Chapter Fourteen

WOMEN AT ALTITUDE

WHEN THE OLYMPIC GAMES were revived in Athens in 1896, a woman named Melopeme trained secretly and — despite the outraged efforts of officials — slipped in to run against and finish with the men. Her achievement was ignored until recently. In 1984 Joan Benoit won the women's Olympic marathon in just half Melopeme's time, which was better than eleven of the last twenty men's Olympic marathon gold medalists. This supremely grueling effort established women's endurance and overcame centuries of discrimination against their participation in "unladylike" sports.

Women had been forbidden to participate in any of the ancient Olympics, being barred even as spectators under pain of death. Instead women had their own Herean Games, honoring the goddess Hera, where their abilities were obvious even though the events were limited. But, whether due to chivalry, idealism, or male chauvinism, or perhaps insecurity, male prejudice continued until 1928 when women were finally allowed to participate in the Olympics, but only after their own Olympics had drawn increasing attention. In the last two decades, for better or worse, the sexual revolution has clearly shown that women can do almost as well as men in most athletic activities (even better in some), and this is substantiated not only in action but by an increasing flow of research.

Men dominated climbing in the Alps during the Golden Age (1850–1875) when most of the great peaks were climbed for the first time, because the culture and mores dictated women's role rather clearly, and few had the courage or audacity to step out of this role. But they were there — for example, the Parminter sisters, whose alpine climbs before 1800 are as unsung as Melopeme's marathon a century later. Maria Paradis (who was sometimes called "Maria of the Mountains") climbed Mont Blanc, at 15,750 feet the highest summit in Europe, in 1808, but two books listing ascents of that beautiful and dangerous mountain do not mention her, and Auldjo, probably the most authoritative, wrote in 1828: "Some years ago a party of guides made the ascent for pleasure. With them was Maria de Mont Blanc, a high-spirited girl."

She may have been seeking publicity for her small creamery, or she may have loved adventure, but never mind: only seven parties had reached the summit before then, and she was the first woman. Though no record of how she felt has survived, a small street in Chamonix is named for her; her little creamery is long gone.

Two English ladies climbed a small mountain near Chamonix, and the queen of Holland made a similar climb. Other women were also interested, though their climbs are not recorded as carefully as those by men. Mrs. Campbell and her daughters made a difficult crossing of a high pass, the Col du Géant, in 1822, bivouacking on the way (for which they were criticized). The guides had difficulties handling the rope, and the women wore long dresses which were a major impediment, but they had a good time and said they would return. Henriette d'Angeville climbed Mont Blanc in 1838 and described her symptoms vividly:

From the base of the Mur de la Côte to the summit I fell into a kind of lethargic sleep which required a halt every ten or twelve steps and an unheard of effort of will to overcome . . . as soon as I sat down a leaden sleep weighed down not only my eyes but all my limbs . . . it was in such a state that I passed the final two hours of the climb, but

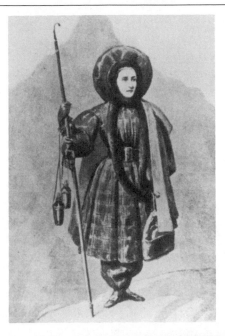

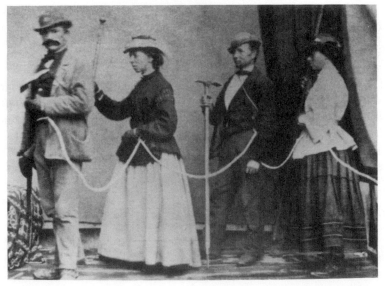

FIGURE 37. EARLY WOMEN CLIMBERS

Maria Paradis was the first woman to climb Mont Blanc and, being a local restaurant owner, probably was not as finely dressed as the next successful woman, Henriette d'Angeville (*shown here, top*) who reached the summit in 1838. The tall alpenstock, with a chamois horn on its end, was standard equipment until early in this century. Fortunately, more sensible, though less dramatic, women's clothing came into common use, though not until after World War II.

The Golden Age of Alpine climbing ran from 1854 to 1885 and among the finest climbers of that glorious period were a few women. Mary Isabella Stratton (*bottom, first on right*) was one of the best: she made the first winter ascent of Mont Blanc and was actively climbing all over the Alps until she was eighty years old. Studio portraits like these were often kept as souvenirs and provide us a nostalgic look at accomplishments, fashions, and relationships in a period which seems much more than a hundred years ago.

---

thought of abandoning the effort never crossed my mind. . . . Once upon the summit my resurrection was immediate; I regained all my mental faculties and was able to enjoy fully the magnificent spectacle.

Her triumph was not disputed, though there were several very different versions of what actually took place, and we read quite different descriptions of her personality and ambitions. Mountain historian Claire Engel called her

. . . a romantic woman longing for glory and excitement; a thwarted maiden lady in her forties, eager to become a society lion, possibly jealous of other well-known women, George Sand for one. . . . She was fascinated by Mont Blanc . . . and pined for years before being able to do as she wished. . . . She had a strange craving for publicity; she wanted glory as a mountaineer, as a writer . . . she thought of going to the bottom of the Channel in a diving bell and in the air in a balloon . . . she was a sort of femme fatale who loved Mont Blanc because she had no one else to love.

Though the lady died before he or Claire Engel was born, R. L. G. Irving, who has written extensively about mountains, was more charitable. According to Irving she was

... a genuine lover of the great mountain. ... She climbed the Olden-horn in her seventieth year. A love of adventure without a trace of the adventuress, a quite remarkable emancipation from convention and a magnificent reserve of strength and determination characterize this vivid personality.

Pikes Peak (1,500 feet lower than Mont Blanc and unglaciated, of course) was not climbed until 1820 — and less than twenty years later the first woman reached the summit. Julia Archibald Holmes, a twenty-year-old bride from Massachusetts, had packed with her wedding finery the "reform" dress of the time, approved by leaders of the suffragette movement. She wrote:

I think an account of my recent trip will be received with some interest by my sisters in reform if not by the rest of mankind since I am perhaps the first who has worn the American costume across that prairie sea which divides the great frontier of the states from the Rocky mountains. ... I wore a calico dress reaching a little below the knee, pants of the same, Indian moccasins on my feet and on my head a hat. ... [The only other woman in the wagon train snubbed her but the men crowded round] ... sometimes gazing at the stove which with its smoke pipe looked quite as much out of place as will the first engine which travels as far away from civilization but oftener they looked on my dress.

Carrying food for six days, "five quilts, a volume of Emerson's essays, and writing materials," she and her husband camped for two days just above the highest spring, where they made a nest of spruce twigs under an overhanging rock and spent a day reading, writing, and admiring the landscape. Next day they reached the top, but cold and a snowstorm kept them from staying long. There Julia read to her husband a verse from Emerson:

> A ready drop of manly blood,
> The surging sea outweighs,
> The world uncertain comes and goes;
> The loser rooted stays.

Julia Archibald deserves more than a footnote in history as one of the early American women climbers, undaunted by the role and habit imposed on them by custom. English ladies were climbing in the Alps, well chaperoned by father or brothers, but even so there were problems. Sleeping in a hut or bivouac when men were present was too shocking to contemplate; instructions where to place the "limbs" could be embarrassing; no mention could be made of toilet. The clothing required of women was restrictive, and few were as bold as Lucy Walker, who shed her crinoline soon after leaving the hotel and is said to have climbed in a red flannel petticoat. She was a strong climber, whatever she wore, and the first woman up the Matterhorn only seven years after it was first climbed. In 1851 "bloomers" were introduced by Amelia Bloomer, a prominent suffragette, but they did not catch on widely for some time.

Mary Isabella Stratton made hundreds of climbs, including four ascents of Mont Blanc (in 1876 the first one in winter). She married a famous guide, Jean Charlet, and together they climbed until she was eighty. Mrs. Edward Buck pioneered many high passes and smaller summits in the second half of the nineteenth century, and by its end women were climbing more and more difficult peaks, but usually with men.

In the last part of the nineteenth century, a few women were going higher than the Alps; of these Annie Peck and Fannie Bullock Workman are the best known. Miss Annie was a professor of Latin and widely recognized as a scholar; she wanted to climb the highest mountain in the Americas because "being always a believer in the equality of the sexes, I felt that any achievement in my line of endeavor would be of advantage to my sex." J. P. Farrar, then editor of the *Alpine Journal*, wrote perhaps with tongue in cheek:

> *I do beg of you, dear lady, to consider well before you exhort your sex to "begin to compete with men in the field of exploration." It may be they will take you too literally and eschew the company of any mere male in their journeys. . . . I am not sure their cares will be lessened thereby, and do consider our loss!*

Miss Annie wore knickerbockers (though they were frowned on) for her climbs in the Andes, proclaiming her belief in women's suffrage, and on her fifth attempt, at age fifty-nine, she climbed Huascaran (22,650 feet high), but was disappointed to find it lower than Aconcagua. I remember meeting her — a tiny, wrenlike lady, erect, bright, interested in everything, though she was well past her eightieth birthday.

Her contemporary, Fannie Bullock Workman, and her husband, a surgeon retired because of a heart condition, claimed the Karakoram as their turf and made an extraordinary series of climbs and journeys through unmapped regions. In the course of eight expeditions they crossed many 20,000-foot passes and camped even higher — at a time when sleeping at such great heights was thought likely to be fatal! Though there is some uncertainty about exactly which peaks they climbed and how high Fannie went, there's no question of this indomitable woman's strength and endurance. She wrote that the local porters suffered from altitude but made no mention of how she and her husband fared. Nor did Annie Peck.

Farrar had been prophetic. Women were already proving that they could do as well as men and the all-women party would soon be common. But first had to come emancipation. Miriam O'Brien (who was to become one of the great alpine climbers, and married a man equally great) wrote of early days:

Isobel and I . . . though we wore with our middy blouses the big full bloomers of the period, considered it more seemly to wear a skirt outside. . . . But that was the beginning and end for me. Trousers . . . were just coming into fashion about the time I needed them. . . . [She had them custom made in Europe.]

A few years later, she was doing formidable climbs in the Alps with one of the leading guides, including the first ascent of two granite needles called the Mademoiselles (and renamed Les Dames Anglais after her climb). In 1930 she was doing "manless climbing" with Alice Damesne, and made one of the more difficult routes on the Grepon, a spectacular pinnacle near Chamonix of which Mummery (who made the first ascent) wrote in 1881:

> *It has frequently been noticed that all mountains appear doomed to pass through three stages: an inaccessible peak — the most difficult climb in the Alps — an easy day for a lady. . . . I must confess that the Grepon has not yet reached this final stage.*

After O'Brien and Damesne had negotiated the famous Mummery crack, one of the great Chamonix guides said sadly:

> *The Grepon has disappeared . . . there are still some rocks standing there, but as a climb it no longer exists. Now that it has been done by two women alone, no self-respecting man can undertake it. A pity too, because it used to be a very good climb.*

Meta Brevoort, Aubrey Le Blond, Freda du Faur are among the many all-but-forgotten names in the history of mountaineering, as are Mary Sheldon, Kate Marsden, Isabella Bishop, and Alexandra David-Neel in the records of difficult and dangerous expeditions to the most remote quarters of the world. Women proved their courage, strength, and endurance, yet it was not until the 1930s that many became part of Himalayan expeditions. By 1960 they were doing increasingly difficult climbs at altitude; in 1975 a Japanese woman and later a Tibetan woman climbed Everest, and many other women have now climbed peaks over 26,000 feet high.

Just as Farrar had facetiously warned, women soon excluded men and made major expeditions to the Himalayas and the Andes. Their spirit was exemplified by one all-women expedition that earned an astronomical sum from the sale of T-shirts boldly labeled "A Woman's Place Is on Top."

Since then women have shown they can often equal what men can do — and this is happily accepted. No one called El Capitan, the magnificent 3,000-foot granite wall in Yosemite, nonexistent because Bev Johnson climbed it solo. Women are regular members of Himalayan expeditions, and it is difficult to tell men from women in summit photos or from the laconic records of many great climbs, where often only first initials are given and mention of a woman may be considered sexist. They have also demonstrated their endurance, ability to accept harsh conditions, and toughness:

In 1974 the tragedy on Pik Lenin in the Pamirs saddened the climbing world when eight Soviet women, the best in the country, died in a terrible storm while camped on the summit; their deaths were due to hypothermia and were made doubly sad because radio contact was continued over the days as one by one died. That they survived as long as they did is a tribute to their endurance and strength of spirit.

In 1984 a man and wife and a Nepalese porter reached 26,000 feet on a great peak; he developed cerebral edema and died soon after a terrible descent to 25,000 feet. She and the Nepalese survived, severely frostbitten; she is alleged to have said later that had he not been so sick she would have gone to the summit alone. Three years earlier the two had nearly perished in a long, severe storm at almost the same spot.

Their natural grace of motion made difficult rock-climbing a natural for women, and when some began leading the most difficult climbs (graded in the United States as 5.11 and 5.12), relying on skill more than strength, resistance to what some saw as intrusion into a man's sport disappeared along with role differentiation. Though unisex clothing, cohabitation, and use of initials and last names blurred external sex differences, it was not thought unmanly when a great climber wept openly at the fatal fall of his friend. Women have been stereotyped as emotional, whereas they may simply be less inhibited in expressing their feelings. To everyone's pleasure some traces of femininity remain: a famous French alpinist (female) said, "I think a woman should remain what is called feminine when going into the mountains, and going to a hairdresser before an important climb is the least I can do."

Most women tend to have less muscle mass than men, but they can double their strength with training without noticeable change in bulk. Though women are almost as strong as men in their trunk and legs, arm strength, even with training, is less than that of men, a fact which is less important when one recognizes that women tend to be lighter and thus have less weight to haul up difficult pitches. We can conclude from all this that well-trained women, with their greater grace and inherent rhythm, and lighter bones and body weight, can climb as efficiently as men, and perhaps even better.

Altitude tolerance and resistance to altitude sickness are the same in men and women. In fact, some data suggest that in the same circumstances, women are less likely than men to develop HAPE or HACE, but statistical proof remains to be established.

Women's pulse rate and blood pressure at altitude are as variable as men's, and there is no agreement as to why. Women's breathing rate and pulmonary ventilation tend to be higher than men's, and thus their ventilatory exchange and alveolar oxygen are perhaps better, but here too the data are scanty. Maximum work capacity in women is less than in men, as a rule, but women can train up as well as men. Like men, those women who start with a higher maximum oxygen uptake at sea level may be better off at altitude, where everyone will function at a percentage of sea level capacity which decreases as altitude increases.

Unlike men, women often have hidden iron deficiency, which becomes more important as the body is called on for more iron to make more red cells as a part of acclimatization. Women seem to be slower in forming red cells during acclimatization, but whether this is due to low iron stores or some other factor is unknown. But if they take supplementary iron, the response to hypoxia improves.

Women who engage in prolonged strenuous physical activity, be it ballet, marathon training, or long mountain expeditions, tend to have scanty menses or even to stop menstruating; this is not a function of altitude but of physical work, and normal cycles resume in time once the strenuous efforts have decreased. But there's a lot of variation among women, some continuing with normal cycles throughout.

Though mountaineering, especially extreme climbs or on the highest mountains, remains a male-dominated sport, women have amply proven they can do almost as well, in technique, in endurance, and in tolerance for altitude. The male chauvinism of several generations ago may have been based on protectiveness, chivalry, territoriality, or simple apprehension that women would beat them at what they felt was their own game. Whatever the reason, discrimination — in climbing at least — is gone for good. We honor Mrs. Tabei and Mrs. Phantong, the first women to climb Everest, not only for this feat, but, with hundreds of other women, for overcoming prejudices and biases and being fully accepted in the world of climbing.

Chapter Fifteen

ON THE SUMMIT

HUMANS SEEM ALWAYS to be trying to set records, as attested by the *Guinness Book of Records,* and each generation seems capable of more than its predecessors. There's only one highest point on earth, though, and when Everest was climbed in 1953, no one could climb higher. But climbing Everest with supplementary oxygen is equivalent to climbing a peak many thousands of feet lower. So the next record would have to be summiting Everest without extra oxygen, and this was done by Rheinhold Messner and Peter Habeler in 1978 — and about a dozen times since. To do so is stretching human capacity to its limit. Or is it? Could we climb higher if there were something higher to climb? There are people at sea level who live with lack of oxygen equivalent to that on the summit of Everest or even higher, because heart or lung disease keeps the oxygen in their blood as low as if they were on the highest mountain.

Soon after the height of Everest was accurately fixed (from a distance) in 1852, speculation began: could man reach the summit and return alive? Some explorers (many of whom left few records) had climbed to 20,000 feet. In 1864 a surveyor and addicted mountaineer, W. H. Johnson, was said to have reached even higher, and twenty years later W. W. Graham claimed to have gotten over 23,000 feet. This was disputed by many, because altitude had killed a number of balloonists who ventured that high. Most of the veteran mountaineers were cautious: few said flatly that reaching such an altitude was impossible — but most doubted it could be done.

As World War II wound down and the altitude training centers were about to be mothballed, I began dreaming of taking men — in a decompression chamber — to a simulated altitude equal to the summit of Everest, protecting them from all the stresses of that high windswept desert and measuring their acclimatization with all the tools available. Fortunately Washington had learned to appreciate the importance of basic research, which contributed so much during the war years, and the climate was hospitable to such a proposal. This was before the great National Institutes of Health had been founded, and research was supported with little formality by private funds or by each of the military services.

It took three months to draw up a plan, win acceptance from command all the way to the Surgeon General, assemble a small team of scientists, find four volunteers, and convert a decompression chamber from a training classroom to a dormitory and laboratory. Under the sympathetic guidance of Captain Ashton Graybiel, head of the Research Division of the School of Aviation Medicine in Pensacola, Florida, Dick Riley and I planned Operation Everest. Lieutenant Commander Margaret Haley took charge of diets and Walter Jarvis and John Patterson carried out many of the studies. In addition to the services of some twenty other naval and civilian personnel already on board, we were given a budget of $1,000 to hire two technicians, Frank Consolazio and George Selden, who rapidly became full members of the team.

The low-pressure chamber was ten feet square and seven feet from floor to ceiling — cramped quarters into which to fit two double-decker bunks, a table, chairs, a bicycle, and each day several working scientists. A heavy steel door separated it from a small antechamber — the lock — which could be taken up and down as needed; this was our elevator. Two huge auxiliary power generators were installed outside the building in case of power failures (not unheard of), crew was trained in emergency procedures, the chamber was refitted, and dozens of other details attended to. A call for volunteers produced several: Horace Hertel, Walter McNutt, Carlton Morris, and Earl Wilkins were selected as subjects. Our official orders (which I wrote) came from Washington:

To obtain data on the respiratory and circulatory changes which occur during acclimatization to altitudes of 25,000 feet and higher. Four subjects would live in a pressure chamber for approximately 20 days during which the chamber would be slowly evacuated to simulate increasing altitude to 25,000 feet or above. Numerous studies would be made at various altitudes.

Operation Everest attracted only amused tolerance when the chamber door was closed on June 27, 1946, for three days of testing at sea level before the simulated ascent started; few understood what we were trying to do — or why. Day after day the pressure was slowly reduced, and each day observers "went up in the lock" to run tests, deliver meals, provide hot baths (in a large barrel), take cardiograms, and draw venous and arterial blood at rest and while the subject was pedalling on a stationary bicycle. In all, 409 lock trips were made, each round trip taking ten to thirty minutes, depending on the altitude.

By the eighteenth day the chamber had reached 18,000 feet; a week later it was at 22,000 feet, where the subjects felt and looked poorly enough to cause us to take the chamber down to 20,000 feet for a few days. Finally on July 30 I wrote:

Things have moved rapidly during the past twenty-four hours. Dr. Riley is having increasing difficulty in placing the needle in our subjects' arteries. . . . At the same time their blood is so thick it clots rapidly in the needle. Too their appetites are very poor and all have lost considerable weight and are feeling much weakened. It is apparent that their time in the chamber is drawing to a close. . . . We have decided to make a "dash for the top" . . . and at 1041 the chamber began its ascent at 1000 feet per hour. . . . I joined the boys for lunch at 22,000 feet taking with me various pieces of apparatus for making

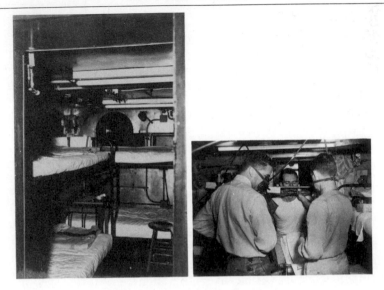

FIGURE 38. OPERATION EVEREST, 1946

During Operation Everest we used equipment that seems primitive compared to what is available today, but nevertheless a great deal of data about acclimatization were obtained. The needles used to draw arterial blood were almost the same as those used twenty years earlier by Barcroft. On the other hand, the respiratory valves, shown here at right, are almost the same as those in use today.

tests and recording observations. The slow ascent continued all through the afternoon. Once an hour each man rode the bicycle for five minutes, meanwhile making comments on his sensations. . . . The atmosphere within and without the chamber was tense. . . . Each thousand feet was more difficult than the preceding one. . . . By the time the chamber reached 26,500 feet at 1611, Wilkins was approaching his peak altitude . . . he was given oxygen. We were all on edge at this crucial point for we had no idea how Wilkins would react when given oxygen. For weeks these men have been starved for oxygen. One of their methods of compensating for lack of oxygen has been to elimi-

nate carbon dioxide, which acts at sea level as the chief stimulus for breathing. The question, then, is what will happen when a man is given pure oxygen in adequate quantities without also being given carbon dioxide. Will he stop breathing since he no longer needs to compensate for lack of oxygen? Will he be intoxicated by the excess of oxygen? Will he notice no change? Wilkins took a few deep breaths of oxygen, his color changed from the deep purple of oxygen lack to a rosy hue. His breathing was normal. He commented on a sense of pressure in his head, and then announced he felt wonderful. . . . The ascent continued. Hertel was next to reach his ceiling . . . at 27,500 feet . . . and asked for oxygen. . . . McNutt and Morris staggered on. As each thousand feet was passed, Morris added a paragraph to a letter he was writing to his family. . . . By 1738 we had reached 28,000 feet where both men were mentally alert, though not capable of strenuous exercise. . . . At 1751 the needle on the altimeter crept up to pass the 29,000 foot mark and reach a maximum of 29,025. Our men were now 23 feet higher than the summit of Everest and they remained at this altitude for twenty-one minutes. Both described their sensations clearly, and expressed pride in their accomplishment.

By then the project had attracted some outstanding physiologists, such as Bruce Dill, John Fulton, Leslie Nims, and some of the navy's top brass; clearly we had a winner. What had we done? From the climber's point of view we had shown that man could reach, and move about, and think on top of the world. We obtained arterial and venous bloods, and alveolar and expired air samples at rest and during and after work on all subjects at several altitudes up to 22,000 feet, and alveolar gas samples every 1,000 feet to the summit, the first ever taken at such heights. X rays showed that the heart actually decreased slightly in size rather than dilating as we feared, and the electrocardiograms showed only a few minor changes. Despite our apprehension (which seems absurd today), the subjects did not stop breathing once the stimulus of oxygen lack was removed when they reached sea level. The published papers from Operation Everest have become a landmark in altitude physiology. Soon after it was over I wrote:

Despite excellent living conditions, adequate food and rest, the four subjects did not acclimatize to altitude either as completely or as rapidly as do mountaineers. The reason for this is not clear, but may be attributed to the confined quarters which made sustained and strenuous exertion impossible. At the higher altitudes the men spent most of their time at rest, and this undoubtedly decreased their work ability just as is the case in a patient confined to bed. Evidence was obtained suggesting that the ability to tolerate high altitudes may depend upon adaptation to low carbon dioxide pressure which results from hyperventilation and in turn raises the arterial oxygen pressure, content and saturation.

In retrospect, it is interesting that we measured altitude in Operation Everest with an aircraft altimeter — the anaeroid type, which is quite accurate but relates pressure to altitude along the standard curve. By that, our subjects had gone to 235 torr pressure — which is 15 to 18 torr lower than the pressure actually measured on the summit of Everest twenty-five years later. Thus the two men had gone to almost 30,000 feet, physiologically.

By 1981 there had been great progress in altitude research: basic concepts had been clarified, a great deal of data had been collected on high mountains, and instrumentation had advanced beyond what we could have dreamed during Operation Everest. It seemed appropriate to try for a repeat study, appropriately enough called Operation Everest II (OEII).

OEII, like its parent, would be an attempt to dissect the marvelous changes the human body undergoes when exposed to lack of oxygen. We know a good deal about these adjustments, and we know a good deal about what happens when the adjustments fail, or when we go to even a modest altitude too fast to allow the changes to develop. What we don't know is which adjustments are due to lack of oxygen per se, and which are caused by the harsh environment at very high altitude. In fact, we aren't completely agreed on which changes are beneficial and which are not. Operation Everest II would again be a study of pure hypoxia, because the subjects would be living in

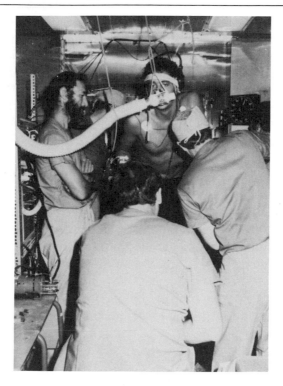

FIGURE 39. OPERATION EVEREST II, 1985

Operation Everest II was very much more complex than its predecessor. For one of the tests, each subject pedaled on a stationary cycle until he was exhausted and could do no more. In other tests, a thin catheter was passed through a vein, into the heart, and from there to the lungs. In this way very accurate measurements of heart action were obtained. Measurements were made at rest and during exercise, and finally during the same exercise while breathing oxygen. We concluded that the summit of Mt. Everest was not the highest point man might be able to reach — if there were anything higher.

a warm, comfortable room, with excellent and ample food and drink, plenty of recreation, opportunity to exercise at any level they wished, and for the most part protected from cold, exhaustion, anxiety, and fear — although some studies would be painful, exhausting, and even frightening.

The subjects were selected from some sixty applicants, as carefully as one should choose members of a major expedition. All were very fit, all were interested in how their bodies functioned, most were climbers, and three had been as high as 20,000 feet or higher. Two were doctors, two were premedical students, and several others had biology or science backgrounds. They were a fantastic group. There was one difference from the subjects in Operation Everest I that we thought might be important: three of the four in the 1946 study smoked continuously in the chamber, but none we chose for 1985 smoked at all.

OEII was far more complicated than the 1946 study: overall, about seventy persons were involved. Instead of three months, it took five years from the birth of the idea to actual start-up. John Sutton, my colleague on the Mt. Logan studies, soon joined the plan, as did John Maher, director of altitude research at ARIEM (the U.S. Army Research Institute of Environmental Medicine), until his untimely death, when Allen Cymerman took his place and John, Allen, and I became the principals.

For some time I had been looking for the right place, and the choice soon became obvious: ARIEM in Natick, Massachusetts. After some persuasion the command agreed to let us use their splendid decompression chamber and excellent laboratory and equipment. Best of all, the army would provide staff to operate chamber and laboratory. Then came four years of frustrating effort to find money — a problem sadly familiar not only to mountaineers but also to researchers. After three requests had been turned down by the National Institutes of Health, and my desperate appeals to many foundations had received only one encouraging response, the chief of the Army

Research and Development Command, General Gary Rapmund, took the project in hand and from then on gave us every consideration — and his enthusiasm, which meant even more. Twenty scientists were invited from among leaders in physiology in the United States and Canada. They were experts in special fields and all were very much involved in altitude research; several were mountaineers as well.

Experiments on humans can only be done after each subject has been thoroughly briefed and understands fully the risks and benefits of every procedure planned; then he must sign a consent form. Before this, every procedure must be approved by a Human Use Review Committee (HURC), a group of medical eagles who look at every aspect not only to protect the subjects, but also to determine what will be learned. We would be doing some rather daring and painful experiments, and getting HURC approval took many months. We would be using sophisticated electronic equipment — and every piece had to be inspected for safety in the chamber. Penetrations had to be drilled through the steel walls for the passage of dozens of shielded wires and tubes. Banks of oxygen cylinders had to be manifolded and fed to many outlets inside the chamber. A proper toilet and shower had to be set in place, a good diet kitchen prepared, and special food obtained. The vacuum pumps and air conditioners would need to run steadily for six weeks: we had to be certain of fallback equipment. We certainly did not anticipate Hurricane Gloria when she hit Natick — but the chamber unit at ARIEM was well prepared and we were able to start only a few days late.

Our goal was to examine all stages of the oxygen transport system during acclimatization to lack of oxygen, as well as the reverse process — the carbon dioxide transport system. We would examine breathing and what drives it while awake and asleep and during maximum work. We would look at the relationship between the ventilation of the lungs and the passage of blood past the lung sacs (alveoli), which is the ventilation–perfusion ratio. We would study muscle metabolism at rest and after violent exertion, and we would examine the many changes which take place in blood during acclimatization.

Retinal photographs were to be taken. Subjects were weighed underwater to determine their percentage of body fat before and after the project, and CAT scans were made for the same purpose. Every bit of food and fluid taken would be recorded to determine why subjects lost weight at altitude — if they did so. Many tests would be run on blood, and bits of muscle would be taken by needle biopsy to measure how muscle uses oxygen at rest and during strenuous work. We were interested in how much work a man could do when acclimatized to very high altitude, and whether he could maintain his normal weight if given plenty of food and comfortable surroundings.

The most ambitious study required passing a small tube (a Swan-Ganz catheter) into an arm vein, to the heart, past its valves, and into the lung. This would enable us to measure many things, among them: blood pressure in the pulmonary artery and in parts of the heart, amount of blood pumped by the heart each minute, and (very important) the amount of oxygen remaining in venous blood returning to the heart from all over the body. We would do another complicated study by injecting a solution containing a number of inert gases to see how fast they cleared the lung by measuring their concentration in expired air. This would give us the diffusing capacity of the lung — the ease or difficulty with which oxygen moves from lung to blood.

The chamber was a little more spacious than that used in 1946. The men would live in the main chamber (twenty by nine feet), which was connected to a small lock (eight by eight), which in turn was attached to a small chamber (nine by twelve), where more tests would be done. In addition to the lock, which served as elevator, there were small pass-through locks in which we could send small items up or down. Lock trips took five to fifteen minutes each way. The chambers were very well ventilated and the levels of oxygen, carbon dioxide, humidity, temperature, and of course barometric pressure in the chamber were continuously recorded. In the lock, accessible to the subjects most of the time, were a toilet and shower. Double-decker bunks, a treadmill, two exercise cycles, and a climbing simulator (Versaclimber, generously loaned to us by the maker) crowded the main chamber and lock, while the small chamber was crammed with instruments of every sort.

Six of the subjects lived for ten days at 25,000 feet and made several trips to 29,000 feet, staying there for as long as four hours. Two subjects were taken out, one at 18,000 and one at 25,000 feet, because of brief collapse blamed on the altitude. Both recovered within minutes. All had headaches beginning about 18,000 feet, but improving above 22,000 feet. All had trouble sleeping, partly due to headache, partly because of very dry, sore throats not helped by anything we could devise, and partly because their periodic (Cheyne-Stokes) breathing kept rousing them from light and restless sleep. All this was very similar to what we had seen in Operation Everest I, and not much different from what was reported on Himalayan expeditions.

Above 20,000 feet their headaches and broken sleep led us to lower the chamber 1,000 to 1,500 feet each night, heeding the traditional doctrine of working high but sleeping low. The ascent profile was quite similar to that of Operation Everest I. We faced a dilemma: if the ascent was too fast, our subjects were less likely to acclimatize fully, but if too slow, the time in the chamber would be unbearably long. By the fortieth day both subjects and scientists felt we had had it!

All of them (and most of the hard-pressed scientists too!) lost weight, about 40 percent of it fat, though all were fit and trim to start with. This was a surprise and disappointment because we went to great lengths to give them the best food we could and catered to every wish (including Ben and Jerry's ice cream — their favorite). They simply lost appetite and took fewer calories. The dietary analysis shows they did have ample minerals and vitamins and plenty of water.

All had been accustomed to lots of exercise, and they continued, running for several hours on the treadmill or cycling against a heavy load, or working out on the Versaclimber (an ingenious device that exercises both arms and legs). But above 20,000 feet they became lethargic, exercised less (though they always felt better when they did so), and took less interest in reading or anything except lying in the sack. They were able to do more, much more, than those who had participated in 1946.

At 25,000 feet they *did* run on the treadmill and they *were* able to work up to a third of their sea level capacity during the maximum exercise test at 25,000 feet, although less at 29,000 feet. When called on, they did have strength — for short bursts of maximum effort. They breathed larger and larger volumes of air during work as altitude increased, and moving air did not seem to be a limiting factor. The amount of blood pumped by the heart at rest and during work decreased as altitude increased, but it did not seem that the ability to move blood limited what they could do.

Alveolar gas samples were taken to measure the amount of oxygen and carbon dioxide deep in the lungs and compare this with the amount in arterial and mixed venous blood. These levels were higher than predicted and blood was not as alkaline as had been predicted by the American Medical Research Expedition to Everest four years earlier.

Could these men have climbed the Hillary step near the top of Everest? Could they have summited and still had some reserve? Only a few have done so without extra oxygen on that mountain. How do the OEII subjects compare with the Everest summiters? Are they physiologically different from you and me, or from Messner, John Roskelly, and many others?

It's important to remember that in 1946 and 1985 we doctors were watching and studying these acclimatizing men with our normal sea level eyes and brains; no one who is unaffected by hypoxia can watch men on top of Everest. Those who have climbed without oxygen have told us that they are close to the limit. They hallucinate, they stagger, they gasp for breath, every step is described as a tremendous effort, the world seems unreal. Our subjects, as we saw them clearly, were not so badly affected.

On the other hand, they were not as well acclimatized as members of an expedition who have spent months on a big mountain. Why, in such a pampered state, did they not acclimatize better? Was ascent too fast, time at altitude too short? Are the stresses of a mountain a help rather than a hindrance in acclimatization? Perhaps the heavy physical work — which the OEII subjects did not do — assists acclimatization more than we anticipated. We don't know.

None of our measurements indicated that they were supermen — just as the tests which have been done on elite summiters show that they excel mainly in will, determination, and ability to endure pain and still press on and up.

Did we learn to predict who will and who will not acclimatize? Did we find any new yardsticks by which to measure acclimatization? Can we predict who will get altitude sickness? As I write this we are not far enough along with number crunching and analysis to answer these important questions. We hope we will be soon.

When all the data have been analyzed and hashed over, we will have some suggestions for mountaineers. Perhaps of more benefit to people in general, we may be able to shine new light on problems faced by the hundreds of thousands of patients who lack oxygen at sea level because of heart and lung disease. For the scientists and the subjects, Operation Everest II remains an unforgettable experience — stimulating, exhausting, overwhelming at times, but very rewarding to all. Asked whether he would do it again, one subject said, "No way . . . no . . . never . . . at least not for a while." That's how we all felt, then.

ALTITUDE AND
BAROMETRIC PRESSURE

WHEN PERIER MADE his tremendous discovery that atmospheric pressure decreased the higher his party climbed on the Puy du Dôme, he was measuring the true atmospheric pressure as shown by his mercury barometer, but this was not necessarily an indicator of the height above sea level, which at that time could not be measured. Today, however, we can make extremely accurate measurements, both of atmospheric pressure and of vertical elevation, which complicates and confuses the reporting of altitude studies. But it's not really as difficult as it seems.

By triangulation, surveyors can measure the vertical distance in feet or meters between mean sea level (average between tides) and the top of a mountain, and we call that its altitude or height above sea level. This is the figure shown on most maps for most mountains.

Atmospheric pressure has been measured very accurately on many mountains and in aircraft and balloons high in the atmosphere, and in very many parts of the world. From these measurements a "standard atmosphere" curve has been drawn which relates vertical distance above sea level to atmospheric pressure under "standard conditions."

However, on top of a mountain, as anywhere else, atmospheric pressure varies with temperature, weather, distance from the equator, and other factors. For example, on an 18,000-foot summit, atmospheric pressure might vary from 405 torr to 370 torr depending on the temperature, season of the year, and latitude. As the atmospheric pressure varied, so of course would the partial pressure of oxygen, since the composition of air is extraordinarily constant and unaffected by altitude, temperature, or weather. Oxygen makes up 20.96 percent of air everywhere, and this percentage of the measured atmospheric pressure tells us the partial pressure of oxygen we breathe. So long as we think of altitude in terms of millimeters of mercury or torr of pressure we are accurately assessing the "physiological altitude" regardless of the number of linear feet or meters above sea level, as Bruce Dill has stated so succinctly. But we need a mercury barometer or we must correct an aircraft altimeter.

Altimeters used by climbers and in aircraft are generally of the aneroid type. In these the altitude is measured by changes in the atmospheric pressure exerted on a small sealed container whose expansion as pressure decreases moves a lever that moves hands indicating the altitude in feet or meters. However, the scale on aneroid barometers and altimeters is derived from the standard pressure–altitude curve and applies only under "standard conditions." The altimeter may show the actual linear feet of elevation, but only under specific conditions and in certain places, and unless corrected it does not (usually) give "physiological altitude." An added complication comes from the fact that the layer of air surrounding the earth is not as thick over the poles as over the equator, and corrections for latitude as well as temperature must be made for reading aneroid barometers. Terris Moore has pointed out that a mountain 29,000 feet above sea level in linear altitude would have a "physiological altitude" equivalent to that of a 26,730-foot summit at 75 degrees north latitude in January, but that of a 30,620-foot summit at 30 degees north latitude in July. He has suggested that the "physiological altitude" on Mt. McKinley is considerably higher, and on Mt. Everest considerably lower than their triangulated height if one measures it as pressure derived from applying the elevation to the standard atmospheric pressure–altitude curve.

Obviously this concerns climbers and pilots who measure their height with altimeters, but should not in any way disturb the conscientious physiologist, who should think of altitude only in terms of millimeters of mercury or torr of atmospheric pressure. For an excellent discussion of this effect see John B. West, S. Lahiri, et al. Barometric pressures at extreme altitudes on Mt. Everest: physiological significance. *Journal of Applied Physiology* 54:1166–1194, 1983.

PEOPLE IN ALTITUDE PHYSIOLOGY

TRYING TO DISCOVER who did what, and when, is one of the most fascinating aspects of research. The deeper you dig, the farther you look, the more likely you are to find unsung heroes — persons whose work precedes, often by many years, that of those now better known. Fame often seems to be capricious in her choice of whom to anoint. Often those whose names have endured are those who sifted the work of others and put together many pieces to make something new and important. Most of us are able to reach however high we do because we stand on the shoulders of those who have gone before.

Here I have noted the names and brief biographies of some great and some obscure persons whose intuition, labor, courage, genius, and ability to bring together the observations of others enabled them to expand our knowledge and our skills. Only a few are here: I omitted those in our century, and regretfully left out many others. Certainly there are many I never found.

ANAXAGORAS (500–428 B.C.) One of the philosophers during the Golden Age of Pericles in Athens, Anaxagoras built on the principles advanced by Empedocles, holding that matter was infinitely divisible, and that all things were held together in an apparently uniform and motionless form. He wrote only one important paper and has not had much permanent impact.

ARISTOTLE (384–322 B.C.) Of all the great philosopher-scientists in the Golden Age of Greece, Aristotle is one of the best known. His scientific concepts were based on logic: he believed the universe to be finite and centered about the earth. Outside of his universe there could be nothing, inside of it there could be no emptiness, i.e., no vacuum. He believed in the four basic elements of fire, air, water, and earth as defined by Empedocles, but rejected the latter's atomic theory. Some consider Aristotle the founder of anatomy because of his studies of the heart and circulatory system. He believed that the pulsation of the heart was due to "boiling" of the blood, which then flowed to the lungs to be cooled. Because of the way he prepared his animals for study, he did not recognize that there were four rather than three chambers in the heart, nor did he distinguish between arteries and veins or recognize the existence of the heart valves. His influence on all of the sciences endured for a thousand years, being challenged successfully only during the Renaissance.

BEECKMAN, ISAAC (1588–1637) Primarily interested in physics, mechanics, and meteorology, he was a progressive thinker, and much concerned with teaching physics and mathematics to the common man. He believed that the universe was infinite, he subscribed to the atomic theory, and he came close to understanding the circulation of the blood. He seems to have understood how pumps worked, and anticipated Torricelli in several theories.

BERNARD, CLAUDE (1813–1878) Although he is one of the best-known physiologists, he was an average student, passing examinations only with difficulty. Fortunately he came under the influence of some of the great physicians of his time, fell in love with physiological experimentation rather than medical practice, and received many honors for his studies of digestive enzymes, liver function, and the autonomic nervous system. He was a great experimenter, and as his studies advanced, his horizons widened and the concept of the constancy of the internal environment became central to most of his experiments and writing. Apparently he was the first to recognize that carbon monoxide killed by replacing oxygen in blood, and he was a pioneer in the study of both toxic and beneficial medications and how they were metabolized. He was the first to recognize the principle of homeostasis — the tendency of living organisms to maintain their own innate stability.

BERT, PAUL (1833–1886) Truly the father of high-altitude physiology, Bert was also a zoologist, a physiologist, and a pioneer in transplant surgery. He was also active and prominent in politics, and his textbooks of natural history, zoology, and the physical sciences were widely printed and translated. Claude Bernard had the greatest influence on Paul Bert and was largely responsible for Bert's major work on barometric pressure. Although less well known than his work at high altitude, his studies of caisson disease (bubble formation in the blood of divers brought up from great depth) were equally innovative. He was primarily a teacher, experimenter, and politician, and never practiced medicine.

BERTI, GASPAR (1600–1643) Although he was primarily interested in astronomy and physics, and a professor of mathematics, Berti's major contribution to science was the apparatus that led to the modern barometer, which he built sometime between 1640 and his death in 1643. None of Berti's own writing has survived, and what we know of his work comes from secondary sources. He did not believe that a vacuum existed above the water column in his crude barometer, because the sound of a bell could be heard ringing in the space, until his friend and biographer Emmanuel Maignan showed him that the sound was transmitted by a metal arm holding the bell! Berti described the device to Torricelli, who made it practical.

BLACK, JOSEPH (1728–1799) In addition to carrying on a busy and distinguished medical practice, Black was a brilliant and popular chemistry teacher, lecturing without notes, demonstrating his experiments with unfailing success, and attracting students from all over the world. His experimental methods were very precise, and he was the first to demonstrate the qualities of carbon dioxide, which he called "fixed air" and recognized as a product of animal metabolism. His experiments with heat were even more important. Black recognized that air was necessary for all forms of combustion, was quite ambiguous in his treatment of the phlogiston theory, and, after Lavoisier's work was known, gradually abandoned the phlogiston theory.

BOERHAAVE, HERMANN (1668–1738) Holding three of the five professorships in the medical school at Leiden, Boerhaave was one of the great teachers of his time, attracting students from all over Europe. He not only lectured for four or five hours a day, but he was also a brilliant bedside teacher and established the modern system of history, physical examination, diagnosis, course of illness, and autopsy. He did not have a clear concept of red blood cells, and his somewhat ambivalent interest in alchemy is indicative of the confusion that still existed in science in Europe during that time. With extraordinary patience, he studied the possibility of transmutation of elements, for example, distilling mercury over 500 times, shaking a sample of mercury continuously for eight and a half months and then distilling it repeatedly, and even boiling one sample of mercury for fifteen and a half years.

BORRICHIUS (BORCH), OLAUS (1626–1690) Borch, a Dane, studied medicine first but became better known as a professor of botany and chemistry. He had a large and busy medical practice and wrote extensively about a wide variety of subjects. In one of his many experiments, he decomposed potassium nitrate to generate oxygen in 1678, but apparently did not pursue the subject.

BOYLE, ROBERT (1627–1691) Born in Ireland, Boyle achieved major influence through his extraordinary work in philosophy, chemistry, physics, and as a founder and principal influence in the Royal Society. Of his wide interests, his best-known work is in the physics of air. He learned of Guericke's air pump, adopted Hooke's design, and confirmed the observations of Torricelli and Berti. He demonstrated that sound could not be transmitted in a vacuum. Boyle studied the behavior of gases, the vacuum, and the properties of matter throughout his life. He supported the concept of atomic structure of all matter, although he used the less specific term *corpuscle*. He was a great experimenter, and described all of his experiments in immense detail so that others might repeat them.

CAVALLO, TIBERIUS (1749–1809) Though born in Italy, Cavallo soon settled in England and took up experimental physics at first with atmospheric electricity, studies inspired by Benjamin Franklin. He then studied the physics of the atmosphere, developed an improved air pump, and wrote a book on the nature and properties of air and "other permanently elastic fluids," as gases were then known. His book *The History and Practice of Aerostation,* which dealt primarily with balloons, is a classic.

CAVENDISH, HENRY (1731–1810) A bachelor who wrote no books and few articles in his long career in natural philosophy, Cavendish was a recluse. Inspired by Newton, he extended the studies made by Black on "fixed air" and heat. He was a firm believer in phlogiston even after Priestley had published his work with oxygen. One of his more extraordinary accomplishments was "the weighing of the world" using a torsion balance, and rounding out Newton's law of gravitation.

CESALPINO, ANDREA (1519–1603) Cesalpino was a philosopher and physician, a follower of Aristotle, and a pioneer in the study of circulation. He realized that the heart pumped blood throughout the body, through the arteries, and received blood from the veins. He described the valves of the heart and pulmonary vessels although he failed to put together a coherent picture of circulation as Harvey later did.

EMPEDOCLES (492–432 B.C.) This early Greek philosopher originated the four-element theory of matter, believing that earth, water, air, and fire were the "roots of all things" and that there were two forces — love and hate — that moved mankind. He believed that animals developed both by chance and by natural selection, and Darwin quoted his work as cited by Aristotle, whom he influenced profoundly. Most of what is known about him is overlaid with legend. He is said to have stopped an epidemic by diverting two rivers, to have changed the climate in a valley by building a wall across a gorge, and to have revived a woman who had been without pulse or respiration for thirty days. His alleged leap into the volcanic crater of Etna may be myth, or impelled by belief in his immortality, or a prank!

GALEN (A.D. 129–199) Few physicians have more profoundly influenced medicine than did this Roman who served as physician to the gladiators after completing twelve years of medical studies. He believed in a "fourfold scheme" which included the four humors of the body, the four elements, the four seasons, the ages of man, and other factors in a harmonious whole. His greatest work was titled *Anatomical Procedures* but was based on observation rather than dissection. He accepted the view of Erasistratus that blood entered the right ventricle from the veins and was prevented from returning by the tricuspid valve. From the right ventricle it went to the lungs by the pulmonary artery and nourished the lungs. He felt that the heart worked like a bellows, actively dilating and passively contracting. He showed that the heart and vessels always contained blood, while Erasistratus had thought that sometimes they could contain air. Galen is best known for his immense pharmacopeia, which dictated medical treatment for many centuries.

GALILEI, GALILEO (1564–1642) His is one of the most famous names in mathematics, physics, and astronomy. He was a firm supporter of Copernicus, and for this he was examined by the Inquisition and condemned to prison, but the sentence was commuted to house arrest for life. His most famous studies were made possible by the thirty-power telescope he developed in 1609, and he is best known for his work in astronomy and in the motions of falling bodies. Galileo treated the existence of a vacuum in a curious way. Having been told that suction pumps and siphons could not lift water beyond a certain height, he explained this with the theory that water had its own inner limited tensile strength, just as a rope or wire will break of its own weight if long enough. He failed to understand that the weight of the atmosphere was the cause of the siphon phenomenon and rejected it even after Giovanni Baliani had clearly explained it to him.

GUERICKE, OTTO VON (1602–1686) Although he was destined for politics and studied law, he became preoccupied by the concept of space and soon became a convert of Copernicus. He wondered about the possibility of a vacuum, how heavenly bodies might affect each other across the emptiness of space, and whether or not space was indeed bounded or limitless. In 1647 he made the first functioning suction pump and ten years later constructed the famous Magdeburg Sphere, which consisted of two hemispheres made of heavy copper, fitted tightly together with a gasket, and then evacuated. The difficulty of separating the evacuated spheres was convincing evidence of the pressure of the atmosphere.

HALES, STEPHEN (1677–1761) Born to an old and distinguished family, Hales took a general education at Cambridge, where he was strongly influenced by Newton's heritage and by the scholarly William Stukeley, but he himself had no formal medical training. Throughout his life he was a clergyman, but his curiosity and ingenuity led him into pioneering studies of blood pressure and circulation for which he was made a member of the Royal Society. At the time the magnitude of the arterial blood pressure was unknown, some contending that it was very large and might actually power muscle contraction. Hales's simple measurement of the arterial blood pressure in a mare ensured him permanent fame, and led him to further studies of the heart, the veins and capillaries, and the mechanics of blood flow. He was very versatile, and his most original — though less known — work involved the force that could raise the sap in plants and trees often to great heights. He demonstrated transpiration, showing that leaves give off not only moisture but also tiny bubbles of gas. This led him to study the gas laws and the composition of air as defined by Hooke, Mayow, and Boyle. He repeated Mayow's experiments, placing either a candle or a small animal under a bell jar and demonstrating that some element in air was consumed before the candle was extinguished or the animal died. Taking this a bit further in a series of rebreathing experiments on himself, he showed that some element of air was consumed and another gas produced by the body, which would not support life. This convinced him that "fresh air" was essential to health and led him to invent ventilators for purifying the air in hospitals and on shipboard, a major advance in public health.

HARVEY, WILLIAM (1578–1657) After receiving his doctorate in medicine at Cambridge, Harvey studied under some of the great anatomists in Italy, returning to London where he became a distinguished physician and an important influence in the Royal College, doing his historic work on circulation in his free time. He had a broad interest in the arts and a wide circle of friends outside of the sciences and was untiring in his studies of the entire animal world, though he is best known for his "discovery" of the action of the heart and circulation. Most of his papers on other areas of natural history were lost in the Great Fire of London. Though Harvey followed Aristotle rather than Galen, his unique contribution came from his ability to put together many theories and observations of others and his own dissections and calculations to produce the first complete and accurate explanation of the coursing of blood through arteries, veins, and tissues, impelled by the heart as a pump. Many others had accurately described parts of the system — Galen's concept of the greater circulation was one bit, and Renaldo Colombo's description of the circulation through the lungs another, but Harvey was the first to make a coherent description of the whole. The logical steps through which he reached his conclusions are fascinatingly revealed in his great book *De Motu Cordis.*

HOOKE, ROBERT (1635–1702) Although described as sickly all of his life, Hooke was a precocious genius whose talents included mathematics, mechanics, and physiology. Before he was eighteen he had mastered geometry and the organ, and described thirty ways of flying, then entered Oxford, where he was befriended by some of the most brilliant men of his time. As assistant to Robert Boyle, he built an improved version of Guericke's air pump, and undoubtedly contributed importantly to formulating Boyle's famous gas laws. By 1660 he had invented a method for using a spring instead of a pendulum to drive a clock, and actually drew up a patent for this, although Christiaan Huygens built the first spring watch in 1674. He joined the Royal Society, becoming curator responsible for several new scientific demonstrations for each weekly meeting. He published his most important book, *Micrographia,* in 1665, containing hundreds of observations made through the newly invented microscope. Less well known are Hooke's studies of air, combustion, and respiration. He showed that the function of breathing was to supply fresh air to the lungs rather than to cool or to pump blood, and along with Mayow, Boyle, and Lower came close to isolating oxygen. He was a tireless inventor, producing brilliant and innovative ideas and a variety of scientific instruments. He was described as a "difficult man in an age of difficult men whose life was punctuated by bitter quarrels which refused to be settled."

HOPPE-SEYLER, ERNST FELIX (1825–1895) Though he was a physician, his major work was in physiological chemistry, a discipline that he really established, editing the first biochemical journal in Germany. He examined the structures of chlorophyll and blood, and obtained hemoglobin in crystalline form for the first time.

IBN AL-NAFIS (1208–1288 approx.) Only in the last thirty years has the work of this great Egyptian physician been rediscovered, and even today his contributions to medicine are inadequately recognized. In his early thirties he planned a comprehensive 300-volume medical text of which eighty volumes were published. Primarily a surgeon, he defined three stages for each operation: diagnosis, during which a patient entrusts the surgeon with his life; the operation; and finally postoperative care. His most extraordinary contribution was his description of the pulmonary circulation in 1242, centuries before Servetus, Colombo, and Harvey. He wrote: *"This is the right cavity of the two cavities of the heart. When the blood in this cavity has become thin, it must be transferred into the left cavity, where the pneuma is generated. But there is no passage between these two cavities, the substance of the heart there being impermeable. It neither contains a visible passage, as some people have thought, nor does it contain an invisible passage which would permit the passage of blood, as Galen thought. The pores of the heart there are compact and the substance of the heart is thick. It must, therefore, be that when the blood has become thin, it is passed into the arterial vein (pulmonary artery) to the lung, in order to be dispersed inside the substance of the lung, and to mix with the air. The finest parts of the blood are then strained, passing into the venous artery (pulmonary vein) reaching the left of the two cavities of the heart, after mixing with the air and becoming fit for the generation of pneuma. . . ."* It is said that his religion and compassion prevented him from dissection, which might have led him to an accurate definition of the total circulation. How widely known his work was during his lifetime is unknown, and whether or not reports of his work reached and influenced his successors is hotly debated.

LAVOISIER, ANTOINE-LAURENT (1743–1794) Although best known for his studies of oxygen (and he is usually credited, erroneously, with having been the first to make it), this Parisian was a distinguished chemist, geologist, and social reformer as well, and it was indeed his activity as a humanitarian and reformer that led to his execution during the Reign of Terror in the French Revolution. In his mid-twenties he first became interested in the properties of air, which led in 1775 to his "discovery" of oxygen, some two years after he had received a letter from Scheele describing how to make that gas. Hales, Black, Priestley, and others were also studying the atmosphere, and although Lavoisier at first knew little of their work, he immediately appreciated the significance of Priestley's work as soon as he learned of it. In 1782–3, following some leads opened by Cavendish and Priestley, Lavoisier showed that water was not a simple material but a combination of "inflammable air" (hydrogen) and "dephlogistigated air" (oxygen). He immediately understood the importance of the Montgolfier balloon ascents in 1783, and during the next two years made a number of hydrogen balloons that rose even better, but his interest in balloons was soon displaced by work on his monumental chemistry textbook, completed only shortly before his death on the guillotine.

LOWER, RICHARD (1631–1691) Lower became one of the most distinguished practitioners of medicine in London and was reported to be the finest English physiologist since Harvey. He became interested in the attempts by Christopher Wren to infuse blood and medication directly into veins, and performed the first successful blood transfusion between dogs in 1665, and between humans in 1667. These studies led to extensive work in cardiopulmonary physiology, and in 1669 he published definitive experiments showing that the bright red color of arterial blood was due to the oxygenation of dark red venous blood during its passage through the lungs. Thus he rounded out Harvey's work and laid the basis for much of what would follow.

MAYOW, JOHN (1643–1679) Born in London and educated at Oxford, Mayow accomplished a great deal in his short life. By the age of twenty-seven he had published two important books on respiration. His studies of the "nitro-aerial spirit" did more than those by others to show that something in air was necessary for, and consumed by, both living animals and a burning candle. He perceived too that this (which a century later was identified as oxygen) entered the blood through the lungs. Some consider Mayow the most important investigator in the distinguished English group who made such advances in the seventeenth century.

MONTGOLFIER, ÉTIENNE (1745–1799)

MONTGOLFIER, JOSEPH (1740–1810) These two brothers were members of a large and prosperous French family engaged in paper manufacture, and both were self-educated in mathematics and science. How or when they became interested in ballooning is unknown, but in 1782 they (and Lavoisier) used hydrogen to fill small balloons of paper or silk to demonstrate the principles of flight, and then turned (probably because hydrogen was scarce and difficult to produce) to hot air. They then constructed a series of increasingly larger balloons using hot air and smoke from moldy hay for lift. Overnight they became world famous and the term *montgolfier* became synonymous with balloons in general, although the brothers themselves made only a few flights. After two years of intense activity both retired to other pursuits, but the science — or sport — they founded endured and spread, bringing notoriety to hundreds of others.

PARACELSUS, THEOPHRASTUS (1493–1541) The real name of this extraordinary man was von Hohenheim. Where or even whether he took formal medical training is unknown, but he did serve as a military surgeon, and he understood that most diseases were of external origin, describing silicosis and tuberculosis as occupational diseases, and recognizing for the first time that syphilis could be congenital. He understood and used the anesthetic and sedative qualities of certain volatile liquids similar to ether, and used mercury and other chemicals as medications. He was a great and pioneering physician, an able chemist, but uncompromisingly destructive toward tradition.

PRIESTLEY, JOSEPH (1733–1804) Since he was educated for the ministry, it is not surprising that Priestley's initial writings were theological discussions of the nature of matter. They aroused great controversy, but throughout all of his work runs a vein of religious conviction that occasionally confuses or obscures his great original contributions. He began to study gases at the age of thirty-seven and became one of the outstanding gas chemists of the world, making many new gases, such as ammonia and sulfur and nitrogen dioxides, and of course working on oxygen. He seems to have cultivated the role of poor scientist in contrast to Lavoisier, with whom his competitive rivalry sharpened with time. In 1770 he began publication of a series of six important books on gases that were widely studied and influential and show a strong influence of Stephen Hales. Priestley's major clash with Lavoisier came over the latter's demonstration of the composition of water and claim for priority in discovering oxygen. Priestley clung to the phlogiston theory even after his voluntary exile to Pennsylvania because of his support of the French Revolution, but his contribution to our knowledge of gases was enormous.

SAUSSURE, HORACE-BÉNÉDICT DE (1740–1799) Although de Saussure is best known for his interest in Mont Blanc, his degree in philosophy from Geneva was in physics, and he was a distinguished mathematician, botanist, and geologist as well. He made studies of the transmission of heat and cold and electricity and magnetism on Mont Blanc as well as observing his own pulse and respirations on all his mountain ascents. His extensive studies of geology, meteorology, and physiology were published in his four-volume work *Voyages dans les Alpes,* a collector's item until reprinted recently. In 1760 he made his first visit to Chamonix and became passionately interested in Mont Blanc, and the reward that he offered to the person who would reach the summit first undoubtedly hastened the ascent.

SCHEELE, CARL WILHELM (1742–1786) Born, educated, and living his entire life in Sweden, Scheele was primarily a pharmacist and chemist whose ingenuity, curiosity, and persistence made him one of the most distinguished scientists of his time. While still under twenty he challenged the phlogiston theory and undertook a series of experiments on plants and animals that convinced him that life was supported by some element in air that was converted in the animal to a gas that would not support life. Although he took voluminous notes, he was slow to publish, and his notebooks have only recently been deciphered. On September 30, 1774, he wrote to thank Lavoisier for one of the latter's books and in his letter gave detailed instructions on how to prepare oxygen, together with basic information on its chemical and physiological properties — the earliest-known written description of oxygen. Scheele knew that some English scientist was following similar studies, and sent to the printer in December 1775 a manuscript in which he described the preparation of oxygen, which would support combustion, and of nitrogen, which would not. Publication was delayed for various reasons, and by the time his book appeared in July 1777, others had published, and credit for Scheele's discoveries went to them. He did important work in both organic and inorganic chemistry, but is almost unknown for his most important contribution.

SCHEUCHZER, JOHANN JAKOB (1672–1733) Born in Switzerland and dedicated to the natural sciences, he practiced medicine, studied mathematics, founded the science of paleontology, and from 1700 onward made many excursions throughout the Alps studying geology, botany, and fossils. He wrote almost 300 books on the history and natural history of Switzerland. His detailed reports of dragons in the Alps, inspired undoubtedly by his interest in fossils, are very interesting but less important than most of his other accomplishments.

SERVETUS, MICHAEL (1511–1553) Servetus was born and first educated in philosophy in Spain, where his religious studies raised in him doubts about the Holy Trinity that made him a fugitive and later led to his execution. He went to France and studied law, where he published his most heretical work for which he was most criticized. He became a proofreader for a publisher, and this aroused interest in medicine, which he studied in Paris, later practicing medicine. His most important book was a theological text in which he described the circulation of the blood from the heart through the pulmonary artery to the lungs and back to the heart. Servetus understood that some "vital spirit" entered the lungs, passed into the blood, and was carried back to the heart and throughout the body. He was on the threshold of comprehending the circulation of the blood, but his text was primarily a religious one, and all but three copies were destroyed when he was burned at the stake for heresy, seventy-five years before Harvey's announcement.

STAHL, GEORG ERNST (1660–1734) Allegedly intolerant and narrow-minded, and undoubtedly controversial, Stahl was an outstanding and active physician and academician, a chemist, and a natural philosopher. He devoted much of his attention to distinguishing between the living and the nonliving and the *anima* that separates them. He preached preventive medicine and felt that doctors had to deal with the entire body and mind rather than individual organs. Strongly influenced by the chemist J. J. Becher, Stahl apparently originated the name *phlogiston* to define combustibility.

Although he recognized that phlogiston and air were related, he believed that phlogiston was an element rather than a quality, and considered carbon as almost pure phlogiston. Although the phlogiston theory was of course wrong, it stimulated much of the essential study that was to follow in the next century.

TORRICELLI, EVANGELISTA (1608–1647) This Italian physicist and mathematician is memorialized in the term "torr," which has recently been used as a measure of barometric pressure. How much he influenced Gaspar Berti's great experiment is unclear, but he had the foresight to see its importance and to use mercury in place of water, thereby making the first true barometer.

GLOSSARY

A-a gradient   The difference in the partial pressure of oxygen and of carbon dioxide between Alveolar air and arterial blood in the lungs.

Acapnia   Literally, no carbon dioxide. Often used to describe a condition in which the partial pressure of carbon dioxide in the blood is lower than normal.

Active transport   The process by which cells "pump" a substance across the cell membrane against a higher concentration.

Altitude   Geographers and cartographers use feet or meters to define height above sea level. Physiologists prefer to express altitude in terms of barometric pressure. *See* "Altitude and Barometric Pressure."

Alveolar   Pertaining to the air sacs in the lung. *See* Alveoli.

Alveoli   The tiny air spaces in the lung where oxygen and carbon dioxide pass between air and blood.

Ambient   The environment surrounding us. Used to refer to air or temperature or humidity.

Anoxemia   Lack of oxygen in blood. *See* Hypoxia.

Anoxia   Lack of oxygen. *See* Hypoxia.

Ataxia   Usually used to describe a staggering gait, but also applies to clumsiness with arms, hands, or fingers. Evidence of neurological disturbance.

Atmospheric   Pertaining to the air that envelops the earth. Usually used to describe pressure or composition of the air.

Barometer   The device developed by Torricelli to measure the weight of the blanket of air that envelops the earth, commonly expressed as torr or millimeters of mercury barometric pressure.

Bronchus   The larger branches of the trachea or windpipe are called bronchi; they subdivide into progressively smaller bronchioles through which air moves in and out of the alveoli.

Buffer   A salt formed by the combination of a weak acid with a strong base (or vice versa) that is able to absorb hydrogen ions with little change in pH (acidity or alkalinity). Buffering power describes the amount of buffer in blood.

Capillaries   Tiny thin-walled vessels which form a network that carries blood from the smallest arteries to the smallest veins and thus enables blood to return to the heart.

Carbon dioxide sensitivity   The responsiveness of the respiratory center to changes in carbon dioxide in the inspired air.

Carbonic anhydrase   An enzyme that facilitates conversion of carbon dioxide to carbonic acid within red cells and to bicarbonate in the kidneys. It is inhibited by acetazolamide (Diamox).

Carboxy-hemoglobin   The compound formed when carbon monoxide attaches to hemoglobin, displacing oxygen.

Carotid   Large artery on each side of the neck supplying the head. Each has a small bulge called the carotid sinus, which monitors blood pressure. A collection of specialized cells adjacent to each artery (the carotid bodies) monitors oxygen in blood.

Carrying capacity   The amount of oxygen that the blood can carry — usually described in volumes percent, i.e., the number of milliliters of gas in 100 milliliters of blood.

Cotton wool spots   Whitish areas seen in the retina of the eye, indicating swelling or edema, without bleeding.

Cyanosis   A bluish color of lips and nailbeds (and in extreme cases, of skin) due to lack of oxygen in the blood, which leaves some of the hemoglobin in the unsaturated form.

Diffusion   The movement of one substance through another, for example, of a gas through a barrier such as a cell wall, or of a dissolved substance throughout the liquid it is dissolved in.

Diuretic   A substance, either natural or synthetic, that increases the formation of urine.

Edema   Fluid that accumulates outside of cells, in the loose tissue between the cells, or within the air sacs (alveoli) of the lungs. Most often seen in feet after standing, or in face and hands after lying down.

Elevation   *See* Altitude.

Hematocrit   The percentage of whole blood occupied by cells (mostly red blood cells). Usually 46 to 50 percent.

Hemoglobin   A complex substance containing four iron atoms (which combine loosely with oxygen), a pigment (which gives blood its color), and a protein (species-specific globin) that determines the type of hemoglobin. Different animals have a metallic ion other than iron, different pigments, and different proteins.

Hypercapnia   Excessive carbon dioxide in blood.

Hypocapnia   Insufficient carbon dioxide in blood. This term is more accurate, though less often used, than "acapnia."

Hypoxia   Lack of oxygen. This has largely replaced the older, less accurate term "anoxia" (literally "no oxygen"). Anoxemia refers to inadequate oxygen in the blood and is used instead of the more precise but clumsy word "hypoxemia."

Hypoxic ventilatory response   The change in rate and/or depth of breathing dictated by a decrease in the partial pressure of oxygen in the inspired air. It is an index of the sensitivity of the respiratory center to oxygen lack.

Intercellular   Between cells.

Interstitial   Pertaining to loose tissue between cells.

Intracellular   Within cells.

Maximal breathing capacity   The largest volume of air one can breathe in one minute.

Maximal oxygen uptake   The largest amount of oxygen one can acquire while working to capacity. It indicates the volume of air one can move, as well as the volume of oxygen passing from lungs to blood and is the standard measurement of fitness and work capacity. Often abbreviated as VO_2Max.

Membrane   A thin molecular covering for cells or organs. The characteristics of a membrane determine its function.

Membrane potential   Each cell membrane has a minute electric charge (bioelectric potential) that maintains the cell's integrity and enables it to fulfill its particular function. Cell death occurs when the membrane potential falls to zero.

Methemoglobin An irreversible form of hemoglobin due to conversion of ferrous to ferric iron, thus interfering with transport of oxygen by red blood cells.

Mitochondria Small bodies within every living cell that perform the functions of that cell. They are the factories of the body and require a large supply of oxygen.

Oxy-hemoglobin The combination of oxygen and hemoglobin, used to describe the dissociation curve relating partial pressure of oxygen to percentage of hemoglobin saturated with oxygen.

Oxygen cascade Shorthand description of the progressive decreases in partial pressure of oxygen as that gas moves from outside (ambient) air into lungs (alveoli), into blood, and finally into the cells, where it is used by the mitochondria.

Oxygen content The amount of oxygen in blood, usually defined as milliliters of oxygen in milliliters of blood. When hemoglobin is fully saturated, oxygen content equals carrying capacity. But when less saturated, capacity is greater than content.

Oxygen transport system Rather loosely used phrase to describe the process of acquisition of oxygen by breathing in, the passage of oxygen from lungs into blood, carriage of oxygen throughout the body by hemoglobin, and finally, passage of oxygen from blood into the cells.

Partial pressure The pressure that one gas in a mixture of gases would exert if it were the only gas present. The number of molecules of the gas present, divided by the total number of molecules, gives the percentage of the gas, and that percentage multiplied by the total pressure of the gas mixture gives the partial pressure. Since we know the percentage of oxygen in air, if we know the barometric pressure, we can easily determine the partial pressure of oxygen at that pressure and thus at that altitude.

Perfusion Flow of blood through tissues or organs, such as the lungs.

Respiration Usually used to describe the process of breathing (inspiration and expiration). Sometimes used to define the entire process of getting and using oxygen. Or, more narrowly, used to refer to the consumption of oxygen and formation of carbon dioxide by cells or tissues.

Respiratory center A collection of highly specialized cells located in the lower part of the brain (the midbrain) that controls the rate and depth of breathing. Primarily controlled by carbon dioxide.

Retina   The layers of nerve tissue, blood vessels, and receptor organs in the back of the eye.

Retinopathy   Abnormalities in the retina, in the case of high altitude, due to increased blood flow and hemorrhages.

Secretion   Formation of a substance by specialized glands. Also used to describe active transport across cell membranes.

Signs and symptoms   Signs are indications that can be seen or heard by an observer; symptoms are sensations perceived only by the individual. The former are objective, the latter are subjective.

Sodium pump   An electrical characteristic of cell membranes that constantly pushes sodium ions out of the cell while retaining potassium ions within the cell. It is one of many "pumps" that maintain proper concentrations of ions within cells by active transport across the membrane.

Torr   *See* Barometer.

Trachea   The windpipe.

Ventilation   Movement of air in and out of the lungs.

Vital capacity   Volume of air in a maximal exhalation after the fullest inspiration. Timed vital capacity refers to the volume that can be exhaled in a specific time, usually thirty seconds or one minute.

VO$_2$Max   *See* Maximal oxygen uptake.

BIBLIOGRAPHY

A BIBLIOGRAPHY IS LIKE a big map: it shows you many of the places where you might want to go, and where you can find directions to other places not shown on the map. No map or bibliography is ever complete. This one, long though it seems, lists only a small fraction of the books and articles relevant to wellness and illness at altitude. But it will lead you to others you may want.

The references I have listed are those that have been most useful and interesting to me, so do not be surprised that many others are omitted. There are more than 32,000 books and articles which deal with hypoxia, high altitude, or closely related subjects. I apologize to those whom I may have overlooked, or who may feel slighted. No two writers would offer the same bibliography.

Only a few papers by some of the leading workers in altitude physiology are listed — but these will lead you to others. Among those who have contributed the most are Cerretelli, Coudert, Dejours, Durand, Grover, Hackett, Hultgren, Kawakami, Kobayashi, Milledge, Pugh, Reeves, Schoene, Severinghaus, Sutton, Ward, and West, but only a few of their papers are cited here. Japanese climber-physiologists are making valuable contributions, but not many of their papers appear in English journals. Few Chinese articles on altitude find their way to the West.

Although this book was written primarily for the nonmedical reader, for the mountaineer, aviator, rescue team, or the thoughtful and inquisitive layman, most of the articles I've cited are in medical journals and may be difficult for the nonprofessional to read — or even to find. That's why I wrote this book in the first place — to translate medispeak into everyday English — and that's why I've written many articles for various mountaineering and nonmedical publications.

Research is properly named: we are constantly searching again — for new evidence, for new understanding of phenomena that for the most part have been searched for and found long ago. Moran Campbell's paper explains this beautifully: in research we are only driving pilings deeper into the swamp, always a little deeper, seldom hitting rock bottom, trying to make a stable platform on which to construct hypotheses and theories.

Without knowledge of what has been done before, a scientist is blind. I hope this book will help others to see where they may wish to go.

BOOKS

Acosta, Joseph. *The Natural and Morall Historie of the East and West Indies.* London: 1604.
Early manuscripts such as this are difficult to find, and I am indebted to Ralph Kellogg for copies of the most interesting portions of this first clear description of the effects of altitude. Other translations call the author José d'Acosta.

Allen, Alexandra. *Travelling Ladies: Victorian Adventuresses.* London: Jupiter Press, 1985.
Brief biographies of eight dauntless female explorers, not including the famous mountaineers, however.

American Alpine Journal. Published in June of each year by the American Alpine Club, 115 East 90th St., New York, NY 10028.

This journal contains a large section describing mountain expeditions in all parts of the world, as well as occasional medical articles. A yearly summary, *Accidents in American Mountaineering*, includes a variety of illnesses and injuries on mountains.

Barcroft, Joseph. *The Respiratory Function of the Blood. Part I. Lessons from High Altitudes.* Cambridge: Cambridge University Press, 1925.

This is one of the classics — an elegant discussion of hemoglobin and oxygen transport at sea level and altitude, as well as of altitude illness and acclimatization.

Baume, Louis. *Sivalaya.* Seattle: The Mountaineers, 1980.

Baume has collected records of all the major Himalayan ascents from the start of Himalayan climbing and in this gives invaluable information about every successful climb and every failure on peaks over 8,000 meters.

de Beer, Gavin. *Early Travellers in the Alps.* London: Sidgwick and Jackson, 1930 and 1966.

This is a fascinating collection of stories of early climbing and traveling in the Alps, with pictures of Scheuchzer's dragons, and stories about Windham, de Saussure, and many others.

Bert, Paul (1877). *Barometric Pressure.* Translated by M. A. and F. A. Hitchcock. Columbus: College Book Co., 1943.

This is the largest collection known of anecdotes, accounts, experiments, and speculations about high altitude. Bert spent years collecting records of mountaineers, explorers, balloonists, and scientific observers. He describes various types of altitude illness, recounts the tragic and humorous experiences of early balloonists, and gives details of hundreds of experiments he performed in pressure chambers and in the laboratory.

Brendel, W., and R. A. Zink, editors. *High Altitude Physiology and Medicine.* New York: Springer Verlag, 1982.

Forty-nine short papers presented at an international symposium dealing with high altitude, in Munich in 1980.

Dill, D. B. *Life, Heat, and Altitude.* Cambridge: Harvard University Press, 1938.

A classic description of the impacts of temperature and oxygen on man.

Dreyfus, Jack. *A Remarkable Medicine Has Been Overlooked.* New York: Simon and Schuster, 1981.

The author presents a highly readable account of diphenylhydantoin (Dilantin) and why he believes it is not widely used. More than 2,000 references are listed, describing the use of Dilantin for many afflictions, including evidence of its effects in hypoxia.

Everest 82. Report of the Soviet Expedition to Everest. Moscow: 1983.

Story of the Soviet climb with some medical data, in Russian.

Folinsbee, Lawrence. *Environmental Stress. Individual Human Adaptations.* New York: Academic Press, 1978.

Frank, Robert G., Jr. *Harvey and the Oxford Physiologists.* Berkeley: University of California Press, 1980.

Frisancho, A. R. *Human Adaptation.* Ann Arbor: University of Michigan Press, 1981.

This is one of the best and most recent books on adaptation and acclimatization to heat, cold, and particularly to altitude.

Gibbs-Smith, C. H. *A History of Flying.* New York: Praeger, 1954.

A complete review of aviation, including a table of dates of importance in aviation from 852 B.C. to A.D. 1953.

Gilbert, Daniel L., editor. *Oxygen and Living Processes.* New York: Springer Verlag, 1981.

Gillespie, Charles C. *Dictionary of Scientific Biography.* New York: Scribners, 1980.

There are sixteen volumes in this fascinating encyclopedia, in which are given biographical and critical sketches of most of the great scientists as far back as we know them. It is difficult not to read like a novel, so well done and so filled with little-known detail are the sketches. A must for anyone interested in the history of science, with a wealth of primary and secondary sources.

————. *The Montgolfier Brothers and the Invention of Aviation, 1783–1784.* Princeton: Princeton University Press, 1983.

This is a new, scholarly book about the first hot-air balloons and how they evolved sufficiently to lift man from the earth. It is a fine companion piece to Robinson's *The Dangerous Sky,* and Gibbs-Smith's *A History of Flying.*

Gribble, Francis. *The Early Mountaineers.* London: T. Fisher Unwin, 1899.

Contains stories about Peter III, Domp Julian, Gesner, Leonardo, and most other early climbers. Describes Gesner's climbing, and the Pontius Pilate legend in detail. Describes Scheuchzer's travels and has several good dragon pictures. The best source of early Alpina.

Hackett, Peter. *Mountain Sickness.* New York: American Alpine Club, 1980.

This is a small (seventy-five pages) handbook dealing with practical aspects of altitude illness as observed in the Himalayas; very useful to take on big mountain expeditions.

Haldane, John S. *Respiration.* New Haven: Yale University Press, 1922; Oxford: Clarendon Press, 1935.

One of the great milestones in our understanding of human respiration.

Hall, W. H. *An Annotated Bibliography of Acute Mountain Sickness.* Natick, MA: U.S. Army Research Institute of Environmental Medicine, 1964.

Twenty-two papers, selected from publications in the last seventy years, are carefully described. Only acute mountain sickness is included. Most of the classic reports are included.

Harvey, William. *De Motu Cordis.* Springfield, IL: Thomas, 1957.

This beautiful translation by Kenneth Franklin contains the Latin text as well, and is the complete text of the famous report that Harvey made in the form of a letter to King Charles and to the Royal College of Physicians describing his experiments, logic, and conclusions. Harvey does not mention the work of his predecessors; though he was certainly aware of what some had done, he almost certainly did not know that Ibn al-Nafis had almost precisely described the circulation four centuries earlier. This is a beautifully detailed and written book.

Health, D., and D. R. Williams. *Man at High Altitude.* London: Churchill Livingstone, 1977.

An excellent and very complete book (290 pages) describing the pathology and physiology of adaptation and maladaptation in mountaineers and permanent residents. Written primarily for scientists, it is intelligible to anyone and a must for doctors interested in altitude. The second edition (1981) has been considerably expanded and brought up to date, though the bibliography has not been noticeably changed.

Hegnauer, S. H., editor. *Biomedicine Problems of High Terrestrial Elevations*. Natick, MA: U.S. Army Research Institute of Environmental Medicine, 1969.
This volume reports a two-day symposium of specialists in various aspects of high altitude.

Henderson, Yandell. *Adventures in Respiration*. Baltimore: Williams and Wilkins, 1939.
Written in a highly readable style, this series of essays describes the early stirrings of research in this century by a friend and colleague of Haldane and Barcroft.

Hooke, Robert. *Philosophical Experiments and Observations*. London: W. and J. Innys, 1676.

Hornbein, Thomas F., editor. *Regulation of Breathing*. New York: Marcel Dekker, 1981.

Houston, Charles S. *High Altitude Physiology Study*. Burlington, VT: Queen City Printers, Inc., 1980.
A collection of forty-four papers published between 1968 and 1980 describing the work of the Arctic Institute High Altitude Physiology Study on Mt. Logan in Canada.

Jaeger, Nicolas. *Carnet de solitude*. Paris: Editions Denoel, 1979.
An extraordinary account (in French) of the author's stay at 6,700 meters (22,000 feet), alone for sixty days, while he made a few physiological and psychological measurements on himself.

Jokl, E., and P. Jokl. *Exercise and Altitude*. Basel: S. Karger, 1968.
An excellent collection of data and theories regarding capability and the constraints on exertion at various altitudes. Of special interest are the chapters on Olympic and Pan-American contests. Excellent reproductions of old photos.

Jourdannet, Denis. *De l'anémie des altitudes et de l'anémie en général, dans ses rapports avec la pression de l'atmosphère*. Paris: Baillier, 1863.

Julyan, R. H. *Mountain Names*. Seattle: The Mountaineers, 1984.

An unusual history of how most of the well-known mountains got their names.

Loeppky, Jack A., and Marvin L. Riedesel, editors. *Oxygen Transport to Human Tissues*. New York: Elsevier Biomedical, 1982.
A collection of thirty talks given at a symposium honoring Dr. Ulrich Luft in Albuquerque, New Mexico, in 1982.

McClung, Jean. *Effects of High Altitude on Human Birth*. Cambridge: Harvard University Press, 1969.

Maughan, J. J., and Kathryn Collins. *The Outdoor Woman's Guide to Sports, Fitness and Nutrition*. Harrisburg, PA: Stackpole Books, 1983.

Medicina de montaña. Proceedings of a Conference on Mountain Medicine, Madrid 1983. Madrid: 1984.
An extensive collection of papers on all aspects of mountain medicine, in Spanish without English translation.

Middleton, Dorothy. *Victorian Lady Travellers*. New York: Dutton, 1965; reprinted Chicago: Academy Chicago, 1982.
Sketches of the best-known traveling explorers of the last century, including Fannie Bullock Workman.

Middleton, W. E. K. *The History of the Barometer*. Baltimore: Johns Hopkins Press, 1964.
This is a detailed scholarly book filled with anecdotes and examples of the first stirring of knowledge about the weight of the atmosphere, the existence of a vacuum, and the evolution of barometers. Middleton deals with Berti's experiments, with the curious Pascal letter, Torricelli, Baliani, and the pioneering observations by Perier on the Puy du Dôme. The last sections deal with modern barometers of various types and sensitivities.

Monge, Carlos. *Acclimatization in the Andes*. Baltimore: Johns Hopkins Press, 1948.
Monge senior was one of the pioneers in altitude research in South America, and this brief discussion of acquired and inherited acclimatization is interesting, though the viewpoint (and bibliography) is almost entirely South American. Monge was first to describe the chronic form of altitude illness that bears his name.

Monge, Carlos, and Carlos Monge, Jr. *High Altitude Diseases*. Springfield, IL: Thomas, 1966.

A brief (ninety-six pages) review of what was known in South America about altitude illness at the time. The bibliography is almost exclusively from South American literature.

Mosso, Angelo. *Life of Man on the High Alps.* London: Fisher Unwin, 1898.
This book, admirably translated by Kiesow from the second Italian edition, is rich with work done on Monte Rosa and in Milan by one of the major explorers of altitude physiology in the nineteenth century.

Mountain Medicine: Proceedings of the University of California Mountain Medicine Symposium, 1983. Davis: University of California, 1983.

Oglesby, Carole. *Women and Sport: From Myth to Reality.* Philadelphia: Lea and Febiger, 1978.

Price, L. W. *Mountains and Man.* San Francisco: University of California, 1981.
An extensive text covering geology, anthropology, biology, and climatology of mountains; exceptional reference material.

Ramsay, William. *The Gases of the Atmosphere.* New York: Macmillan, 1902.
A fascinating collection of anecdotes and experiments done by Boyle, Priestley, Cavendish, Scheele, and others, written by the man who isolated argon.

Richalet, J. P., editor. *Médecine de l'alpinisme.* Paris: Masson, 1984.
Review (in French) of mountain medicine with special attention to altitude illness, hypothermia, and accidents.

Ringebach, G. *L'Adaptation à l'altitude et le mal des montagnes.* Paris: Maloine, 1983.
A summary (in French) of current knowledge and understanding of high-altitude physiology and clinical mountain sickness. Of special value is the bibliography, which includes 550 references, many of them not known in this country.

Rivolier, J., P. Cerretelli, et al. *High Altitude Deterioration.* New York: Karger, 1985.
Proceedings of the International Symposium on High Altitude and Cold Injury held in Chamonix, France, in March 1984.

Robinson, Douglas H. *The Dangerous Sky.* Seattle: University of Washington Press, 1974.

An excellent history of man's attempts to fly, including a great deal of information about lack of oxygen in aviation.

Schmidt-Nielsen, Knut. *Animal Physiology: Adaptation and Environment.* London: Cambridge University Press, 1979.

This is a fascinating and delightfully written text that deals with comparative physiology in all sorts of animals. Filled with illustrations, it gives the average reader insight into the myriad ways organisms learn to live in different environments.

Seghers, Carroll. *The Peak Experience: Hiking and Climbing for Women.* New York: Bobbs-Merrill, 1979.

Sutton, J. R., C. S. Houston, and N. L. Jones, editors. *Hypoxia, Exercise, and Altitude.* New York: Alan R. Liss, 1984.

This Proceedings of the Third Hypoxia Symposium (1983) in Banff is a valuable collection of papers on cold, work, altitude, and their interrelationships.

Sutton, J. S., editor. *Seminars in Respiratory Medicine: Man at Altitude.* Vol. 5, No. 2. New York: Thieme-Stratton, 1983.

This issue devotes over 150 pages to articles about various aspects of altitude acclimatization and illness. An important source.

Sutton, John, Norman Jones, and Charles Houston, editors. *Hypoxia: Man at Altitude.* New York: Thieme-Stratton, 1982.

Thirty-eight papers and many abstracts presented at the Second International Hypoxia Symposium at Banff in 1981 deal with the effects of hypoxia from many causes, with case reports of several episodes of mountain illnesses.

Underhill, Miriam. *Give Me the Hills.* New York: Methuen, 1956.

One of the most delightful books about women climbers in the early twentieth century, written by an outstanding mountaineer.

Van Liere, E. J., and J. C. Stickney. *Anoxia, Its Effects on the Body.* Chicago: University of Chicago Press, 1962.

First published in 1942, this is a complete inventory of the effects of oxygen lack on various organs and systems of the body and probably the richest source of bibliography to that date; the edition of 1962 is a reprint rather than an updated revision of an invaluable work.

Ward, M. *Mountain Medicine.* London: Crosby Lockwood, Staples, 1975.

This is an encyclopedia of all aspects of mountain medicine, including altitude, cold, sun, illness, and injury. Written in a staccato summary style, it is most useful as a reference.

West, J. B. *Everest the Testing Place.* New York: McGraw Hill, 1985.

A pleasantly informal account of the American Medical Research Expedition to Everest, written from one individual's point of view, with a chapter summarizing the scientific results, and a transcript of the summit radio transmission and tapes.

―――. *Respiratory Physiology.* Baltimore: Williams and Wilkins, 1974.

The most compact and readable book on how the lungs work and how oxygen is transferred to and by blood. Many diagrams and tables. Deals mainly with normal physiology and thus is an essential basic work in understanding altitude illness. Easily readable by nonphysicians.

West, J. B., and S. Lahiri, editors. *High Altitude and Man.* Bethesda, MD: American Physiological Society, 1983.

A collection of many of the publications of the American Medical Research Expedition to Everest in 1981.

West, John B., editor. *High Altitude Physiology.* Stroudsburg, PA: Hutchinson Ross, 1981.

Most of the important papers in high-altitude physiology going back to Acosta are collected in this useful book, one of the Benchmark series of classic papers in physiology.

Wulff, L. Y., I. A. Braden, F. H. Shillito, and J. F. Tomashefski. *Physiological Factors Relating to Terrestrial Altitudes.* Columbus: Ohio State University Press, 1968.

A collection of some 4,000 references relating to many types of high-altitude problems. Though not annotated, it is a valuable resource book.

PAPERS

Abelson, A. Altitude and fertility. *Human Biology* 48:83–92, 1976.

Abelson, A., P. T. Baker, et al. Altitude, migration, and fertility in the Andes. *Population Biology* 21:12, 1974.

Aberman, A., C. M. Fulop, et al. The metabolic and respiratory acidosis of acute pulmonary edema. *Annals of Internal Medicine* 76:173–84, 1972.

Albert, R. K., et al. Leukotriene C4 and D4 increase pulmonary vascular permeability in excised rabbit lungs. *Chest* 83:85S, 1983.

Ali, J., and L. D. H. Wood. Pulmonary vascular effects of furosemide on gas exchange in pulmonary edema. *Journal of Applied Physiology* 57:160–67, 1984.

Altschule, M. D. Acute pulmonary edema: pitfalls in diagnosis and treatment. *Medical Counterpoint,* pp. 11–17, July 1969.

Alzamora-Castro, V., G. Garido-lecca, et al. Pulmonary edema of high altitude. *American Journal of Cardiology* 7:769–78, 1961.
One of the earliest complete clinical papers, reporting twenty-seven cases of high-altitude pulmonary edema in valuable detail. Often overlooked.

Arias-Stella, J., and H. Kruger. Pathology of high altitude pulmonary edema. *Archives of Pathology* 76:147–57, 1963.
The first detailed autopsy report (two cases) of high-altitude pulmonary edema, emphasizing (erroneously) the role of a hyaline membrane.

Austin, F., C. M. Carmichael, et al. Neurological manifestations of chronic pulmonary insufficiency. *New England Journal of Medicine* 257:580–90, 1957.

Avery, M. E., and I. D. Frantz. To breathe or not to breathe? What have we learned about apneic spells and sudden infant death syndrome? *New England Journal of Medicine* 309:107–8, 1983.

Baier, H., et al. Ventilatory drive in normal man during semistarvation. *Chest* 85:225, 1984.

Baker, P. T. Human adaptation to high altitude. *Science* 163:1149–56, 1969.

Balasubramanian, V., V. Kaushik, et al. Effects of high altitude hypoxia on left ventricular systolic time intervals in man. *British Heart Journal* 37:272–76, 1975.

Barbashova, Z. Cellular level of adaptation. In *Handbook of Physiology,* section 4:37–57, edited by D. B. Dill, E. F. Adolph, and

C. G. Wilber. Washington, D.C.: American Physiological Society, 1964.

This is a thought-provoking analysis of the "struggle" responses which enable survival during hypoxia, while the "adaptive" changes have time to mature.

Barcroft, J., A. Cooke, et al. The flow of oxygen through the pulmonary epithelium. *Journal of Physiology* 53:450, 1920.

In this classic paper, Barcroft describes definitive experiments which proved that oxygen passed from lungs to blood by simple diffusion, thus putting an end to the secretion theory. Especially interesting from a historical point of view is the account of arterial sampling for the first time in altitude research.

Bernard, G. R., and K. L. Bingham. Pulmonary emboli: pathophysiologic mechanisms and new approaches to therapy. *Chest* 89:594–601, 1986.

Berry, D. T. H., et al. Sleep apnea syndrome: a critical review of the apnea index as a diagnostic criterion. *Chest* 86:529, 1984.

Berssenbrugge, A. D., et al. Effects of sleep state on ventilatory acclimatization to hypoxia in humans. *Journal of Applied Physiology* 57:1089, 1984.

Birmingham Medical Research Expeditionary Society. Acetazolamide in control of acute mountain sickness. *Lancet,* p. 180, January 24, 1981.

Confirmed the value of acetazolamide in preventing acute mountain sickness during an expedition to the Andes.

Bisgard, G. E., M. A. Busch, et al. Ventilatory acclimatization is not dependent on cerebral hypocapnic alkalosis. *Journal of Applied Physiology* 60:1011–15, 1986.

Bixler, E. O., A. Kales, et al. Sleep apneic activity in older healthy subjects. *Journal of Applied Physiology* 58:1597–1601, 1985.

Blesa, M. I., S. Lahiri, et al. Normalization of blunted ventilatory response to acute hypoxia in congenital cyanotic heart disease. *New England Journal of Medicine* 296:237–41, 1977.

The ventilatory response to breathing low oxygen was blunted (made smaller) in young children born with heart defects, but when these defects were corrected, the children responded normally to low oxygen, showing that a blunted HVR is reversible.

Block, A. J. Is snoring a risk factor? *Chest* 10:525, 1981.
A brief editorial discussing the nighttime hypoxia caused by severe snoring and its long-term effects on health.

Block, A. J., P. Boysen, et al. Sleep apnea, hypopnea and oxygen desaturation in normal subjects. *New England Journal of Medicine* 300:513–18, 1979.

Boyer, S. Endurance test on Colorado's 14,000 foot peaks. *Summit* 24:30–35, February–March, 1978.
Description of a remarkable series of climbs in which two men averaged 7,000 vertical feet daily for twenty-one days, climbing all fifty-four of the 14,000-foot peaks in Colorado.

Boyer, S. T., and F. D. Blume. Weight loss and changes in body composition at high altitude. *Journal of Applied Physiology* 57:1580–85, 1984.

Boylen, C. T., D. W. Cugell, et al. Continuous or nocturnal oxygen therapy in hypoxemic chronic obstructive pulmonary disease. *Annals of Internal Medicine* 93:391–98, 1980.

Bradley, B. L., A. E. Garner, et al. Oxygen assisted exercise in chronic obstructive lung disease. *American Review of Respiratory Disease* 118:239–42, 1978.

Braun, S. The prevalence and determinants of nutritional changes in chronic obstructive pulmonary disease. *Chest* 86:558, 1984.
In these sixty outpatients with COPD, weight loss was associated with inadequate caloric intake. Arterial oxygen levels were not measured but the authors say the role of hypoxemia has not been established.

Broughton, J. O., and T. C. Kennedy. Interpretation of arterial blood gases by computer. *Chest* 85:148–49, 1984.

Burki, N. K. Effects of acute exposure to high altitude on ventilatory drive and respiratory pattern. *Journal of Applied Physiology* 561:1027–31, 1984.

———. Arterial blood gas measurement. *Chest* 88:3–4, 1985.

Busch, M. A., G. E. Bisgard, et al. Ventilatory acclimatization to hypoxia is not dependent on arterial hypoxemia. *Journal of Applied Physiology* 58:1874–80, 1985.

In goats, lack of oxygen to the body and to the brain is not necessary for developing hyperventilation.

Campbell, E. J. M. Clinical science. *Clinical Science and Molecular Biology* 51:1, 1976.
The annual lecture of the Medical Research Society (Canada) is wise and witty and rich in insights into the relationships between medical research and practice.

Carlson, R. W., R. C. Schaeffer, et al. Edema fluid and coagulation changes during fulminant pulmonary edema. *Chest* 79:43–49, 1981.

Castellini, M. A., B. J. Murphy, et al. Potentially conflicting metabolic demands of diving and exercise in seals. *Journal of Applied Physiology* 58:392–99, 1985.
A brief but intriguing discussion of how certain diving mammals reconcile the demands for oxygen by muscular exertion with the apnea which occurs during prolonged dives.

Cerretelli, P. Limiting factors to oxygen transport on Mt. Everest. *Journal of Applied Physiology* 40:658–67, 1976.

Child, G. On Broad Peak. *Mountain* 94:18–21, 1983–84.
A graphic, moving account of the death of Dr. Pete Thexton from altitude illness during an alpine-style attack on this peak. Lessons for everyone.

Clark, C. F., R. K. Heaton, et al. Neurophysiological functioning after prolonged high altitude exposure in mountaineering. *Aviation, Space and Environmental Medicine* 54:203–07, 1983.

Claude, A. The coming of age of the cell. *Science* 189:433–36, 1974.
This was Claude's acceptance speech when he was awarded the Nobel Prize for Medicine or Physiology and is a beautifully written, almost lyrical description of what was known about the cell at that time.

Claybaugh, J. R., et al. Antidiuretic responses to eucapnic and hypocapnic hypoxia in humans. *Journal of Applied Physiology* 53:815–23, 1982.

Colice, G. L., and G. Ramirez. Effect of hypoxemia on the renin-angiotensin-aldosterone system in humans. *Journal of Applied Physiology* 58:714–30, 1985.

This is a brief but clear discussion of the complicated relationships of these hormones in men breathing low-oxygen gas mixtures for one hour.

Cooper, K. R., et al. Effect of short-term sleep loss on breathing. *Journal of Applied Physiology* 53:855, 1982.
Sleep loss causes significant deterioration in ventilation, which may be important in patients with lung disease.

Cotev, S., J. Lee, et al. The effects of acetazolamide on cerebral blood flow and cerebral tissue PO_2. *Anesthesiology* 29:471–77, 1968.

Cournand, A. The historical development of the concepts of pulmonary circulation. In *Pulmonary Circulation,* edited by W. R. Adams and I. Veith. New York: Grune and Stratton, 1959.
A beautifully written and scholarly history of circulation to the lungs from the year A.D. 150 to 1900. Invaluable source materials.

Crawford, R. D., and J. W. Severinghaus. CSF pH and ventilatory acclimatization to altitude. *Journal of Applied Physiology* 45:275–83, 1978.

Cudaback, D. D. Effect of altitude on performance and health at 4km telescopes. *Publications of the Astronomical Society of the Pacific* 96:463–510, 1984.

Cudkowicz, L., H. Spielvogel, et al. Respiratory studies in women at high altitude. *Respiration* 29:393–426, 1972.

Cusick, P., O. Benson, et al. Effect of anoxia and high concentrations of oxygen on the retinal vessels: preliminary report. *Staff Meetings of the Mayo Clinic* 15:500–02, 1940.

Cystic Fibrosis Foundation. Airline travel for children with chronic pulmonary disease. *Pediatrics* 57, 1976.
Interesting discussion of cabin pressures and risks for children with chronic lung disease.

D'Alonzo, G. E., et al. Differentiation of patients with primary and thromboembolic pulmonary hypertension. *Chest* 85:457, 1984.

Davies, H., and N. Gazetopoulos. Dyspnea in cyanotic congenital heart disease. *British Heart Journal* 27:28–41.
This is a comprehensive study of twenty patients with a variety of congenital heart problems, at rest and during exercise. Arterial oxy-

gen was measured by saturations that ranged from 97 percent to 54 percent; calculated arterial PO_2 ranged from 59 to 29 torr at rest, and fell to 27 to 14 torr with exercise. Ages ranged from fifteen to forty-one years. One patient dropped oxygen saturation to 20 percent but continued to exercise until stopped because of cyanosis.

de Bold, A. J. Atrial natriuretic factor: a hormone produced by the heart. *Science* 230:767–70, 1985.

Dejours, P. Mount Everest and beyond: breathing air. In *A Companion to Animal Physiology,* edited by C. R. Taylor, et al. Cambridge: Cambridge University Press, 1982.

Dempsey, J. A. Is the lung built for exercise? *Medicine and Science in Sports and Exercise* 18:143–55, 1986.

Dempsey, L., J. O'Donnell, et al. Carbon monoxide retinopathy. *American Journal of Ophthalmology* 82:692–93, 1976.

Dickinson, J., D. Heath, et al. Altitude-related deaths in seven trekkers in the Himalayas. *Thorax* 38:646–56, 1983.

Dill, D. B. Physiological adjustments to altitude changes. *Journal of the American Medical Association* 205:123, 1968.
This is a concise summary of the changes in all parts of the oxygen transport system responsive to hypoxia, written by one of our great contemporaries.

Dill, D. B., and D. S. Evans. Report barometric pressure! *Journal of Applied Physiology* 29:914–16, 1970.
A brief, authoritative discussion of variations in barometric pressure due to weather, latitude, and season. Important pressure altitude data are included.

Drinkwater, B. L. Response of women mountaineers to maximal exercise during hypoxia. *Aviation, Space and Environmental Medicine* 50:657–62, 1979.

Drinkwater, B. L., P. O. Kramar, et al. Women at altitude: cardiovascular response to altitude. *Aviation, Space and Environmental Medicine* 53:472–77, 1982.

Eastman, J. Mount Everest in utero. President's address. *American Journal of Obstetrics and Gynecology* 64:701, 1954.

Eckman, M., A. L. Barach, et al. Effect of diet on altitude tolerance. *Journal of Aviation Medicine* 16:328–40, 1945.

Editorial. Pulmonary oedema of high altitude. *Lancet,* pp. 309–10, February 10, 1962.

Editorial. Pulmonary oedema of mountains. *British Medical Journal,* pp. 65–66 (and letters pp. 231–32), July 8, 1972.

Editorial. Exercise oedema. *Lancet,* p. 961, May 5, 1979.

Editorial. Vasodilator therapy for pulmonary hypertensive disorders. *Chest* 85:145–46, 1984.

Elliott, P.R., and H. A. Atterbom. Comparison of exercise response of males and females during acute exposure to hypobaria. *Aviation, Space and Environmental Medicine* 49:415–18, 1978.

Escourrou, P., D. G. Johnson, et al. Hypoxemia increases plasma catecholamine concentrations in exercising humans. *Journal of Applied Physiology* 57:1507–11, 1984.

Farrukh, I. S., J. R. Michael, et al. Thromboxane induced pulmonary vasoconstriction: involvement of calcium. *Journal of Applied Physiology* 58:34–44, 1985.
Though these studies were done on rabbits, the data may apply to man.

Faulkner, J. A., J. T. Daniels, et al. Effects of training at moderate altitude on physical performance capacity. *Journal of Applied Physiology* 26:85–87, 1967.

Faulkner, J. A., J. Kolias, et al. Maximum aerobic capacity and running performance at altitude. *Journal of Applied Physiology* 24:685–91, 1968.

Federal Drug Administration Bulletin, Vol. 13, No. 3, 1983.
Describes certification of acetazolamide for prevention of acute mountain sickness.

Fein, I. A., and E. C. Backow. Neurogenic pulmonary edema. *Chest* 81:318–20, 1982.

Filley, G., G. Swanson, et al. Chemical breathing controls: slow, intermediate, and fast. *Clinics in Chest Medicine* 1:13–32, 1980.

Finch, C., and C. Lenfant. Oxygen transport in man. *New England Journal of Medicine* 286:407–15, 1972.
This is one of the basic papers defining the entire oxygen transport system and has stood the test of time.

Fishman, A. R. Brain edema. *New England Journal of Medicine* 293:706–7, 1975.

Fitzgerald, M. P. The changes in breathing and the blood at various altitudes. *Philosophical Transactions of the Royal Society, Series B* 203:351–71, 1913.
This is the complete report of this young woman's pioneering studies of alveolar air at a time when few women were daring such efforts.

Fitzgerald, R. S. The respiratory control system. *Chest* 85:585, 1984.

Flenley, D. C. Clinical hypoxia: causes, consequences, and correction. *Lancet,* pp. 542–46, March 11, 1978.
Valuable concise summary of the clinical aspects of hypoxia in patients at sea level.

Folinsbee, L. J., J. A. Wagner, et al., editors. *Environmental Stress: Individual Human Adaptations.* New York: Academic Press, 1978.
Contains several chapters on women in athletic contests and at altitude.

Folkman, J. Angioneogenesis: initiation and control. *Annals of the New York Academy of Science* 401:212–26, 1982.

Forwand, S., M. Landowne, et al. Effects of acetazolamide on acute mountain sickness. *New England Journal of Medicine* 279:839–41, 1968.
This is one of the first, if not the first, carefully controlled studies to demonstrate the benefits of acetazolamide (Diamox) in prevention of mountain sickness.

Frand, U. I., C. S. Shim, et al. Heroin-induced pulmonary edema. *Annals of Internal Medicine* 77:29–35, 1972.

Frayser, R. F., C. S. Houston, et al. Retinal hemorrhage at high altitude. *New England Journal of Medicine* 282:1183–85, 1970.
The first detailed report of the incidence of retinopathy at high altitude, after which came the larger Mt. Logan studies.

―――. The response of the retinal circulation to high altitude. *Archives of Internal Medicine* 127:708–12, 1971.
In this follow-up paper is a description of the dilatation and tortuosity of retinal vessels at high altitude, together with calculations of the rate of blood flow in the eye.

Fred, H. L., A. M. Schmidt, et al. Acute pulmonary edema of altitude: clinical and physiological observations. *Circulation* 25:929–37, 1962.

Genton, E., et al. Alterations in blood coagulation at high altitude. In *Hypoxia, High Altitude, and the Heart.* Basel: Karger, 1970.

Getts, A. G., and H. Hill. Sudden infant death syndrome: incidence at various altitudes. *Developments in Medical Child Neurology* 24:64–68, 1982.

Gilbert, D. L. The first documented description of mountain sickness: the China story. *Respiration Physiology* 52:315–26, 1983.

———. The first documented description of mountain sickness: the Andean or Pariacaca story. *Respiration Physiology* 52:327–47, 1983.

Githens, J. H., C. R. Phillips, et al. Effects of altitude on persons with sickle hemoglobinopathies. *Rocky Mountain Medical Journal* 72:505–9, 1975.

Glynn, L. M., et al. The sodium pump. *Annual Review of Physiology* 37:13, 1975.

Goldberg, N. M., J. P. Dorman, et al. Altitude-related splenic infarction in sickle cell trait — Case reports of a father and son. *Western Journal of Medicine* 143:670–2, 1985.

Gong, H., D. P. Tashkin, et al. Hypoxia-altitude simulation test. *American Review of Respiratory Disease* 130:980–86, 1984.
This paper suggests that patients with chronic lung disease be given a simulated altitude test, breathing down to 13.9 percent oxygen, to predict how they will tolerate air travel.

Graham, W. G. B., and C. S. Houston. Short-term adaptation to moderate altitude in patients with chronic obstructive lung disease. *Journal of the American Medical Association* 240:1491–94, 1978.

Grant, I., R. K. Heaton, et al. Brain dysfunction in COPD. *Chest* 77:2, 1980.
These authors show that patients with hypoxia due to COPD have neurophysiologic deficits suggestive of organic brain dysfunction.

Gray, G. Studies on altitude illness with special reference to high altitude pulmonary edema. Doctoral thesis, University of Toronto, Institute of Medical Science, 1976.

An extensive, scholarly review of the various theories of etiology of high-altitude pulmonary edema, with special attention to the concept of platelet microemboli.

Green, C., J. Butts, et al. The relationship of anoxic susceptibility to diet. *Journal of Aviation Medicine* 16:328–40, 1945.

Green, J. F., M. Shelton, et al. Alveolar-to-arterial PCO_2 differences. *Journal of Applied Physiology* 54:349–54, 1983.

Greene, M. K., et al. Acetazolamide in prevention of acute mountain sickness: a double-blind controlled cross-over study. *British Medical Journal* 283:811, 1981.

A well-designed study of twenty-four persons climbing in Kenya; acetazolamide was effective in preventing acute mountain sickness.

Gronbeck, C. Chronic mountain sickness at an elevation of 2000 meters. *Chest* 85:577, 1984.

This poorly documented single-case report is unfortunately likely to be quoted often. The data presented do not support the diagnosis.

Grover, R. F. Speculations on the pathogenesis of high altitude pulmonary edema. In *Advances in Cardiology* 57:1, edited by J. H. K. Vogel. Basel: Karger, 1980.

Grover, R. F., H. N. Hultgren, et al. Pathogenesis of acute pulmonary edema at high altitude. *Central Hemodynamics and Gas Exchange,* pp. 409–20, 1971.

Grover, R. F., and J. T. Reeves. Oxygen transport in man during hypoxia. High altitude compared with chronic lung disease. *Bulletin of European Physiopathology of Respiration* 15:121–33, 1979.

An important paper in which the authors conclude that high-altitude hypoxia elicits different responses than does hypoxia due to chronic lung disease.

Hackett, P. H., and I. D. B. Rennie. Rales, peripheral edema, retinal hemorrhage and acute mountain sickness. *American Journal of Medicine* 67:214–18, 1979.

Report of a clinical study of 200 trekkers in the Mt. Everest region. Pulmonary rales were noted in 23 percent, edema in 18 percent, and retinal hemorrhages in 4 percent. Half of those who flew to 9,000 feet and a third of those who walked to that altitude experienced mountain sickness at 14,000 feet.

Hackett, P., I. D. B. Rennie, et al. The incidence, importance and prophylaxis of acute mountain sickness. *Lancet,* pp. 1149–55, November 27, 1976.

Hackett, P. H., R. B. Schoene, et al. Acetazolamide and exercise in sojourners to 6,300 meters — a preliminary study. *Medicine and Science in Sports and Exercise* 17:593–97, 1983.

Haldane, J., A. Kellas, et al. Experiments on acclimatization to reduced atmospheric pressure. *Journal of Physiology* 53:185–95, 1920.

Hanley, D. F. Health problems at the Olympic Games. *Journal of the American Medical Association* 221:987–90, 1972.

Hannon, J. P. Alterations in serum electrolyte levels in women during high altitude (4300 m) acclimatization. *International Journal of Biometrics* 14:201–9, 1970.

———. Nutritional aspects of high altitude exposure in women. *American Journal of Clinical Nutrition* 29:604–13, 1976.

Hansen, J. P., and W. A. Evans. A hypothesis regarding the pathophysiology of acute mountain sickness. *Archives of Environmental Health* 21:666–69, 1970.

Hansen, J. P., L. H. Hartley, et al. Arterial oxygen increase by high carbohydrate diet at altitude. *Journal of Applied Physiology* 33:441–45, 1972.

Hara, M. A renaissance of high altitude mountaineering. *Iwa To Yuki,* Tokyo, no date.

Heath, D. Hypoxia and the pulmonary circulation. *Journal of Clinical Pathology* 79:30S, 11–21, 1979.

Hedemark, L. L., and R. S. Kronenberg. Ventilatory and heart rate responses to hypoxia and hypercapnia during sleep in adults. *Journal of Applied Physiology* 53:307–12, 1982.

Heffner, J. E., et al. Platelet induced pulmonary hypertension and edema. *Chest* 83:78S, 1983.

Henderson, Y. The last thousand feet on Everest. *Nature* 3631:921–23, 1939.

Hepburn, M. L. The influence of high altitude in mountaineering. *Alpine Journal* 20:368–93, May 1901.

A valuable review of eighteenth- and nineteenth-century accounts of altitude sickness and the theories then current. Hepburn suggests that a man following certain dietary, training, and breathing routines can climb to 30,000 feet without oxygen. On pages 438–40 Sir Martin Conway, a great mountaineer, comments on the paper and mentions the importance of "years of acclimatization." Other distinguished climbers added good comments.

———. Some reasons why the science of altitude-illness is still in its infancy. *Alpine Journal* 21:161–79, August 1902.

Continuation and expansion of his talk the year before. Here he discusses the various theories in detail. Together the two papers are a thorough review of the "state of the art" at the start of our century.

Hill, N. S. Case records of the Massachusetts General Hospital. *New England Journal of Medicine* 313:1003–12, 1985.

An important case describing the development of chronic pulmonary artery hypertension due to multiple pulmonary embolism over a period of five years.

Holzell, T. Oxygen use on Mt. Everest. *Summit* 31:20–28, March–April 1985.

An authoritative review of the various types of oxygen equipment available and practical for climbers today.

Hornbein, T. R. Response to "acute mountain sickness — type R." *Summit* 23:33–35, October–November 1977.

The controversy over the value of Rolaids as a preventive for mountain sickness as experienced on Mt. Rainier is discussed and the author demonstrates that Rolaids do not have value in AMS.

Horrobin, D. F. High altitude pulmonary edema. *East African Medical Journal,* pp. 327–31, 1972.

Houston, C. S. Operation Everest, a study of acclimatization to anoxia. *Naval Medical Bulletin* 46:12–24, 1946.
Summary description of Operation Everest.

———. Acute pulmonary edema of high altitude. *New England Journal of Medicine* 263:478–80, 1960.

The first contemporary account of high-altitude pulmonary edema.

————. Altitude illness — 1976 version, and High Altitude Physiology Study on Mt. Logan. *American Alpine Journal* 20:407–28, 1976.

————. Lessons from high altitude pulmonary edema. *Chest* 74:399–400, 1978.

————. Altitude illness — recent advances in knowledge. *American Alpine Journal* 22:153–59, 1979.

————. The quest to understand high altitude: a trip back in time and a look ahead. *Postgraduate Medicine* 73:307–14, 1983.

————. Altitude illness. In *Emergency Clinics of North America* 2:503, 1984.

————. Migraine and altitude headache. *Summit* 31:30, September–October 1985, and 31:30, November–December, 1985.

————. Incidence of acute mountain sickness. *American Alpine Journal* 27:162–65, 1985.

————. High altitude pulmonary edema. In *Current Pulmonology* 7:227–40, edited by Daniel H. Simmons. Chicago: Year Book Publishers, 1986.
A review of current concept of etiology, concluding that HAPE is a high permeability, high pressure edema. Extensive references.

————. Operation Everest II: A study of acclimatization to extreme altitude. In press 1986.

Houston, C. S., and R. L. Riley. Respiratory and circulatory changes during acclimatization to high altitude. *American Journal of Physiology* 149:565–88, 1947.
Detailed pulmonary and arterial studies made during a thirty-five-day low-pressure-chamber study of acclimatization.

Huang, S. V., et al. Hypocapnia and sustained hypoxia blunt ventilation on arrival at high altitude. *Journal of Applied Physiology* 56:602, 1984.

Hudgel, D. W., R. J. Martin, et al. Contribution of hypoventilation to sleep oxygen desaturation in chronic obstructive pulmonary disease. *Journal of Applied Physiology* 55:669–77, 1983.

————. Mechanism of arterial oxygen desaturation during sleep in COPD. *Chest* 85:30S, Supplement, 1984.

Hultgren, H. N. Treatment and prevention of high altitude pulmonary edema. *American Alpine Journal* 14:363–72, 1965.

————. Reduction of systemic blood pressure at high altitude. In *Hypoxia, High Altitude and the Heart.* Basel: Karger, 1970.

Hultgren, H. N., and R. F. Grover. Circulatory adaptation to high altitude. *Annual Review of Medicine* 10:119–52, 1968.

Hultgren, H. N., R. F. Grover, et al. Abnormal circulatory responses to high altitude in subjects with a previous history of high altitude pulmonary edema. *Circulation* 44:759–70, 1971.

Hultgren, H. N., C. E. Lopez, et al. Physiologic studies of pulmonary edema at high altitude. *Circulation* 29:393–408, 1964.

Hultgren, H. N., and E. A. Marticorena. High altitude pulmonary edema: epidemiological observations in Peru. *Chest* 74:372–76, 1978.

Hultgren, H. N., W. Spickard, et al. High altitude pulmonary edema. *Medicine* 40:289–300, 1961.
This early article describes eighteen patients with pulmonary edema at 12,000 feet in the Andes and thirteen suggestive cases in mountaineers. The literature is reviewed and possible mechanisms discussed. Fifteen of the eighteen cases in the Andes developed HAPE after return to altitude following a brief stay at sea level. An important early paper.

————. Further studies of high altitude pulmonary edema. *British Heart Journal* 24:95–192, 1962.

Hurtado, A. Physiological and pathological aspects of life at altitude. Rimac, Lima, Peru (privately translated from the Spanish for Houston).
A dissertation given at the time of Hurtado's induction into the Faculty of Medicine, containing detailed clinical and pathological data on five cases of maladaptation. One of the five may be a case of high-altitude pulmonary edema, but the other four are less clear. Though not available in English, this paper is most frequently cited as the initial clinical description of HAPE.

———. Some clinical aspects of life at high altitudes. *Annals of Internal Medicine* 53:247–55, 1960.

Hyers, T., C. Scoggin, et al. Accentuated hypoxemia at high altitude in subjects susceptible to high altitude pulmonary edema. *Journal of Applied Physiology* 46:41–46, 1979.
Seven high-altitude residents considered to be HAPE–susceptible were compared with nine low-altitude residents without a history of HAPE, in a twelve-hour decompression-chamber stay at 13,500 feet.

Hyman, A. L., et al. Vasodilator therapy for pulmonary hypertensive disorders. *Chest* 85:145, 1984.

Jackson, F. The radiology of acute pulmonary edema. *British Heart Journal* 13:503–18, 1951.

Jaeger, J. J., J. T. Sylvester, et al. Evidence for increased intrathoracic fluid in man at high altitude. *Journal of Applied Physiology* 47:670–76, 1977.

Japanese Journal of Mountain Medicine. A recent arrival in mountain medicine presents some different ideas and views in English summaries and covers many important altitude problems.

Jennett, S. Snoring and its treatment. *British Medical Journal* 289:335, 1984.

Johnson, T. S., et al. Prevention of acute mountain sickness by dexamethasone. *New England Journal of Medicine* 310:683, 1984.
In a double-blind cross-over study, eight men were given dexamethasone or placebo and taken rapidly to 15,000 feet in a decompression chamber. They remained for forty-two hours and those given dexamethasone had significantly fewer symptoms than those given placebo. Similar results have since been obtained on Mt. McKinley.

Jones, D. P., et al. Intracellular oxygen supply during hypoxia. *American Journal of Physiology* 243:247–53, 1982.

Jones, J. B., S. C. Wilhoit, et al. Oxyhemoglobin saturation during sleep in subjects with and without the obesity-hypoventilation syndrome. *Chest* 40:9–15, 1985.
An interesting discussion of what used to be called Pickwickian syndrome, known today as alveolar-hypoventilation.

Jouty, Sylvain. The history of altitude. *Alpine Journal* 86:90–95, 1981.

Juratsch, C. E., R. F. Grover, et al. Reversal of pulmonary vaso-constriction induced by main pulmonary arterial distention. *Journal of Applied Physiology* 58:1107–14, 1985.

Karliner, J. S., F. F. Sarnquist, et al. The electrocardiogram at extreme altitude: experience on Mt. Everest. *American Heart Journal* 109:505–13, 1985.
Report of minimal electrocardiographic changes found during the American Research Expedition to Mt. Everest in 1981.

Kawakami, Y., F. Kehi, et al. Relation of oxygen delivery, mixed venous oxygenation, and pulmonary hemodynamics to prognosis in chronic obstructive pulmonary disease. *New England Journal of Medicine* 308:1045–49, 1983.

Kellogg, R. H. Effect of altitude on respiratory regulation. *Annals of the New York Academy of Science* 109:815–28, 1963.

———. Altitude acclimatization: a historical introduction emphasizing the regulation of breathing. *The Physiologist* 11:37–57, 1966.
A scholarly and delightful discussion comparing the old with the modern understanding of acclimatization.

———. La pression barométrique: Paul Bert's hypoxia theory and its critics. *Respiratory Physiology* 34:1–8, 1978.

Kleiner, J. P. High altitude pulmonary edema. *Journal of the American Medical Association* 234:491–95, 1975.

Koo, K., et al. Arterial blood gases and pH during sleep in chronic obstructive lung disease. *American Journal of Medicine* 58:663–70, 1975.

Kramar, P. O., and B. L. Drinkwater. Women on Anapurna. *Physician and Sportsmedicine* 8:1–7, March 1980.

Kramar, P. O., B. L. Drinkwater, et al. Ocular functions and incidence of acute mountain sickness in women at altitude. *Aviation, Space and Environmental Medicine* 54:116–20, 1983.

Kronenberg, R. S., et al. Pulmonary artery pressure and alveolar gas exchange in man during acclimatization to 12,470 feet. *Journal of Clinical Investigation* 50:827, 1971.

This pioneering study examined pulmonary artery pressures in four men during seventy-two hours at 12,470 feet and three others during five days in which they walked four miles to 14,255 feet and back.

Kryger, M. Breathing at high altitude: lessons learned and application to hypoxemia at sea level. *Advances in Cardiology* 27:11, 1980.

LaBelle, J. C. High-altitude research atop Canada's highest peak. *American Alpine Journal* 17:96–104, 1970.

Lahiri, S., and J. S. Milledge. Muscular exercise in the Himalayan high altitude residents. *Proceedings of the Federation of American Societies of Experimental Biology* 58:663–70, 1975.

Lane, P. A., and J. H. Githens. Splenic syndrome at mountain altitudes in sickle cell trait. *Journal of the American Medical Association* 253:2251–54, 1985.

Lange, V. Diamox — a potential aid in acclimatization. *Climbing* 84:58, June 1984.

Larragh, J. H. Atrial natriuretic hormone. The renin-aldosterone axis, and blood pressure–electrolyte homeostasis. *New England Journal of Medicine* 313:1330–40, 1985.

Larson, E. B., et al. Acute mountain sickness and acetazolamide. *Journal of the American Medical Association* 248:328, 1982.
A randomized trial of acetazolamide in sixty-four climbers on Mt. Rainier.

Lassen, N. A., D. Ingvar, et al. Brain function and blood flow. *Scientific American* 239:62–71, 1978.

Lee, B. C., H. V. Zee, et al. Site of pulmonary edema after unilateral microembolization. *Journal of Applied Physiology* 47:556–60, 1979.
Dogs in whom one lung was embolized by micro-glass beads showed accumulation of fluid in the embolized lung; the authors conclude that this is evidence that release of local factors increased permeability.

Lehninger, A. L. How cells transform energy. *Scientific American,* pp. 62–82, September 1961.

Lenfant, C., and K. Sullivan. Adaptation to high altitude. *New England Journal of Medicine* 284:1298–1310, 1971.
This is one of the modern classics in altitude physiology as it relates to acclimatization. Many references.

Lesch, M., G. J. Caranasos, et al. Controlled study comparing ethacrynic acid and mercaptomerin in the treatment of acute pulmonary edema. *New England Journal of Medicine* 279:115–22, 1968.

Lilienthal, J., and R. L. Riley. An experimental analysis in man of the oxygen pressure gradients from alveolar air to arterial blood during rest and exercise at sea level and at altitude. *American Journal of Physiology* 147:199–205, 1946.

Long, I. D. Sickle cell trait and aviation. *Aviation, Space and Environmental Medicine* 53:1021–29, 1982.

McFarland, R. A. Psychophysiological implications of life at altitude, including the role of oxygen in the process of aging. In *Physiological Adaptations: Desert and Mountain,* edited by M. K. Yousef, S. M. Horvath, and H. W. Bullard. New York: Academic Press, 1972.

McKechnie, J. K., W. P. Leary, et al. Acute pulmonary edema in two athletes during a 90-km running race. *South African Medical Journal* 56:261–65, 1979.

Maher, J. T., L. G. Jones, et al. Effects of high altitude exposure on submaximal endurance capacity of man. *Journal of Applied Physiology* 37:895–98, 1974.

Mahoney, B. S., and J. Githens. Sickling crises and altitude. *Clinical Pediatrics* 18:431–38, 1979.

Maresh, C. M., B. J. Noble, et al. Maximal exercise during hypobaric hypoxia (477 torr) in moderate altitude natives. *Medicine and Science in Sports and Exercise* 16:360–67, 1983.

Marticorena, E. Evaluation of therapeutic methods in high altitude pulmonary edema. *American Journal of Cardiology* 43:308–12, 1979.

Marticorena, E., F. A. Tapia, et al. Pulmonary edema by ascending to high altitudes. *Diseases of the Chest* 43:273–83, 1964.

Mason, G. R., and R. M. Effros. Flow of edema fluid into pulmonary airways. *Journal of Applied Physiology* 55:1262–68, 1983.

Massaro, D. Oxygen: toxicity and tolerance. *Hospital Practice,* pp. 96–100, July 15, 1986.

Matthews, B. The physiology of man at high altitudes. *Proceedings of the Royal Society of London* 143:1–4, 1954.

Meehan, R. T., et al. The pathophysiology of high altitude illness. *American Journal of Medicine* 73:395–403, 1982.

Meerson, F. Z. Role of synthesis of nucleic acids and protein in adaptation to the external environment. *Physiological Reviews* 55:79–125, 1975.
A masterful review of the major changes made at the cellular level to adjust or adapt to a changed external environment.

Menitove, S. M., et al. Oxygen rebreathing and exercise responses in humans. *Journal of Applied Physiology* 56:1039, 1984.

Menon, N. D. High altitude pulmonary edema. *New England Journal of Medicine* 273:66–74, 1965.

Michael, C., K. W. Khoo, et al. Factors inducing periodic breathing in humans: a general model. *Journal of Applied Physiology* 53:644–59, 1982.

Miles, D. S., et al. Absolute and relative work capacity in women at 758, 586, and 523 torr barometric pressure. *Aviation, Space and Environmental Medicine* 51:439–44, 1980.

Milledge, J. S. Acute mountain sickness. *Thorax* 38:641–45, 1983.

———. The great oxygen secretion controversy. *Lancet,* pp. 1408–11, February 22, 1985.
A brief but fascinating discussion of the debate between Barcroft and Haldane over the question: Does the lung actively secrete oxygen at high altitude?

Mitzner, W., and J. T. Sylvester. Hypoxic vasoconstriction and fluid filtration in pig lungs. *Journal of Applied Physiology* 51:1065–71, 1981.

Monge, C. High altitude disease. *Archives of Internal Medicine* 59:32–40, 1937.

Monroe, C. G. Mountain sickness. *Alpine Journal* 16:446–55, August 1893.
Detailed discussion of the various theories of mountain sickness current at the time; Monroe believed that "spinal anemia" was the major cause.

Moore, L. G., et al. The incidence of pregnancy-induced hypertension is increased among Colorado residents at high altitude. *American Journal of Obstetrics and Gynecology* 144:423–29, 1982.

————. Variable inhibition by falling CO_2 of hypoxic ventilatory response in humans. *Journal of Applied Physiology* 56:207, 1984.

Moore, L. G., P. Brodeur, et al. Maternal hypoxic ventilatory response, ventilation, and infant birth weight at 4,300 m. *Journal of Applied Physiology* 60:1401–6, 1986.

Moore, T. The world's great mountains: not the height you think. *American Alpine Journal* 16:109, 1968.
A discussion of barometric pressure variations due to latitude, climate, and temperature, including speculations about variations in physiological altitude on Mt. McKinley and Mt. Everest.

Mordes, J. P., et al. High altitude pituitary-thyroid dysfunction on Mount Everest. *New England Journal of Medicine* 308:1133–38, 1983.

Mortimer, E. A., R. R. Monson, et al. Reduction in mortality from coronary heart disease in men residing at high altitude. *New England Journal of Medicine* 296:581–85, 1977.

Moss, G. Shock, cerebral hypoxia, and pulmonary vascular control. *Bulletin of the New York Academy of Medicine,* 1973.
This is the most complete report of Moss's cross-transfusion experiments and seems to show that cerebral hypoxia alone can cause pulmonary edema even when the lungs are normally oxygenated.

Murray, R. H. S., S. Shropshire, et al. Attempted acclimatization by vigorous exercise during periodic exposure to simulated altitude. *Journal of Sports Medicine and Physical Fitness* 3:135–42, 1968.

National Institutes of Health. *Report of Workshop on Arachidonic Acid Metabolites and the Pulmonary Circulation.* Bethesda, MD: National Institutes of Health, 1982.

A concise and complete review of substances released in the lung blood vessels and their effect on flow and pressure and permeability.

Neumann, P. H., C. M. Kivlen, et al. Effect of alveolar hypoxia on regional pulmonary perfusion. *Journal of Applied Physiology* 56:338–42, 1984.

Noble, W. H. Pulmonary edema: a review. *Canadian Anaesthetic Society Journal* 27:286–300, 1980.

Noble, W. H., J. C. Kay, et al. Reappraisal of extravascular lung thermal volume as a measure of pulmonary edema. *Journal of Applied Physiology* 48:120–29, 1980.

Oelz, O., H. Howald, et al. Physiological profile of world-class high altitude climbers. *Journal of Applied Physiology* 60:1734–42, 1986.

An important study done by a large group of climber-physiologists, showing that the best high-altitude climbers have slightly greater stimulus to breathe at altitude, but are otherwise not very different from ordinary people, except in the crucial characteristics of courage, stoicism, and determination.

Olivart, M. T., et al. Hemodynamic effects of nifedipine at rest and during exercise in primary pulmonary hypertension. *Chest* 84:14, 1983.

Onal, E., J. A. Leech, et al. Relationship between pulmonary function and sleep-induced respiratory abnormalities. *Chest* 87:437–41, 1985.

Orr, W. C. Sleep-related breathing disorders: an update. *Chest* 84:475–80, 1983.

A good review of recent work in sleep and breathing, snoring, and apnea with many references.

———. Sleep apnea, hypoxemia, and cardiac arrhythmias. *Chest* 89:1–2, 1986.

Oscal, L. B., B. T. Williams, et al. Effect of exercise on blood volume. *Journal of Applied Physiology* 24:622–24, 1968.

Owens, G. R., R. M. Rogers, et al. The diffusing capacity as a predictor of arterial oxygen desaturation during exercise in patients with chronic obstructive pulmonary disease. *New England Journal of Medicine* 310:1218–21, 1984.

Pease, A. Mountain climbing in antiquity. *Appalachia* 33:289–98, 1961.
This is a charming short review of many of the most unusual and interesting tales of man's attitude toward mountains in the dim past.

Pemberton, L. B. Shock lung with massive tracheal loss of plasma. *Journal of the American Medical Association* 237:2511–14, 1977.

Penberthy, L. Acute mountain sickness — type R. *Bulletin of Mountain Safety Research.* Seattle: Mountain Safety Research, Inc., 1976.

Perkins, J. F. Historical development of respiratory physiology. Introduction to *Handbook of Physiology,* section 3, volume 1, edited by W. O. Fenn and H. Rahn. Washington, DC: American Physiological Society, 1964.
A superb review of the evolution of what we know about respiratory physiology, from the time of Plato to 1930. Indispensable for those interested in the history of medicine.

Perutz, M. Hemoglobin structure and respiratory transport. *Scientific American* 239:92–122, 1979.
A scholarly and understandable description of hemoglobin and how it binds to and releases oxygen in man and some animals.

Phillips, J. F., H. L. Nieman, et al. Noncardiac causes of pulmonary edema. *Journal of the American Medical Association* 234:531–32, 1975.

Phillipson, E. Regulation of breathing during sleep. *American Review of Respiratory Disease* 115:217–24, 1977.

Pizzo, C. Eye problems and mountaineering: prevention and treatment. *Climbing* 90:61, 1985.

Pugh, L. G. C. Muscular exercise on Mount Everest. *Journal of Physiology* 141:233–61, 1958.

———. Physiological and medical aspects of the Himalayan scientific and mountaineering expedition 1960–61. *British Medical Journal* 2:621–29, 1962.
Summary of observations made during five months at 19,000 feet, including many resting and exercising studies never done at altitude

before. This classic expedition — "Silver Hut" — set the stage for future high-mountain scientific research.

Pugh, L. G. C., and M. P. Ward. Some effects of high altitude on man. *Alpine Journal* 61:507–520, 1957.
An important summary of the 1951 Everest reconnaissance, the 1952 Cho Oyu scientific party, and the successful ascent of Everest in 1953, discussing all aspects of altitude and man in nontechnical terms. Many astute comments and observations.

Rahn, H., H. T. Bahnson, et al. Adaptation to high altitude: changes breath-holding time. *Journal of Applied Physiology* 6:154–57, 1953.

Ravenhill, T. Some experiences of mountain sickness in the Andes. *Journal of Tropical Medicine and Hygiene* 20:313–20, 1913.
This appears to be the first detailed description of the various forms of altitude illness as we classify them today: AMS, HAPE, and HACE. It is a classic description of clinical observations made when Ravenhill was a mining company physician in a remote station. No references. Reproduced in West's *High Altitude Physiology,* q.v.

Reed, D., and R. H. Kellogg. Changes in respiratory response to CO_2 during natural sleep at sea level and at altitude. *Journal of Applied Physiology* 13:325–30, 1958.

Reeves, J. T., et al. Physiological effects of high altitude on the pulmonary circulation. In *Environmental Physiology III,* Vol. 20. Baltimore: University Press, 1979.
State-of-the-art review of changes in flow, pressure, permeability, and release of vaso-active substances in the blood vessels of the lung in man exposed to high altitude.

Reeves, J. T., L. G. Moore, et al. Headache at high altitude is not related to internal carotid arterial blood velocity. *Journal of Applied Physiology* 59:909–15, 1985.
The concept that altitude headache is a function of the rush of blood to the brain seems to be refuted in this study, though cerebral blood pressure was not (and cannot yet be) measured accurately.

Reeves, J. T., W. W. Wagner, et al. Physiological effects of high altitude on the pulmonary circulation. *International Review of Physiology* 20:289–304, 1979.

Refsum, H. E., et al. Serum electrolyte, fluid and acid-base balance after prolonged heavy exercise at low environmental temperature. *Scandinavian Journal of Clinical and Laboratory Investigation* 32:117, 1973.
This unique study of forty-one men before and after a 90-km cross-country ski race at 0 degrees centigrade, running for nine hours, showed remarkably small changes in electrolytes, glucose, and other serum components.

Reihman, D. H., M. O. Farber, et al. Effect of hypoxemia on sodium and water excretion in chronic obstructive lung disease. *American Journal of Medicine* 76:87–94, 1984.

Reinhard, J. High altitude archaeology and Andean mountain gods. *American Alpine Journal* 25:54–67, 1983.

Reite, M., et al. Sleep physiology at high altitude. *Electro-encephalography and Clinical Neurophysiology* 38:463–71, 1975.

Rennie, I. D. B., and J. Morrissey. Retinal changes in Himalayan climbers. *Archives of Ophthalmology* 93:395–400, 1975.

Robertson, J. D. The membrane of the living cell. *Scientific American,* 5–20, April 1962.

Robin, E. D. Of men and mitochondria: coping with hypoxic dysoxia. *American Review of Respiratory Diseases* 122:517–31, 1980.
An engaging and stimulating discussion of how severe hypoxia is managed in patients at sea level. A case of Tetralogy of Fallot with an arterial PO_2 of 35 is discussed.

Robin, E. D., C. E. Cross, et al. Pulmonary edema. *New England Journal of Medicine* 288:239–49, and 292–304, 1973.
Comprehensive review, in two parts, of all types of pulmonary edema.

Roth, E. Sickle cell gene in evolution: solitary wanderer or a nomad in a caravan of interacting genes. *Journal of the American Medical Association* 253:2259–60, 1985.

Rounds, S. Pulmonary hypertensive diseases. *Chest* 85:397–403, 1984.

Roy, S. Circulatory and ventilatory effects of high altitude acclimatization and deacclimatization of Indian soldiers — a prospective study 1964–72. New Delhi: General Printing Company, undated.

This booklet contains a large amount of data describing the cardiac and pulmonary changes in troops both rapidly and slowly exposed to high altitude, as well as in residents at the same and higher altitudes. The report is somewhat marred by numerous typographical and mathematical errors.

Ruch, T., H. D. Patton, et al. In *Neurophysiology*. Philadelphia: Saunders, 1965.

Russell, Count Henry. On mountains and mountaineering in general. *Alpine Journal* 5:241, November 1871.
Lovely article with a few paragraphs about altitude illness as it was then perceived.

Ryn, Zdzislaw. Nervous system and altitude syndrome in high altitude asthenia. *Acta Medica Polska* 22:2–28, 1979.
This is a short version of a large manuscript describing the emotional and neurological condition of forty Polish mountaineers before, during, and after several expeditions to very high altitude. Although many of the subjects had severe injuries, illness, or emotional breakdowns, thus making it difficult to attribute their problems to hypoxia alone, Ryn concludes that prolonged exposure to extreme altitude may leave permanent effects.

Schneider, E. Physiological effects of altitude. *Physiological Reviews* 1:631–59, 1921.
This is one of the more complete discussions of what was known about altitude illness and acclimatization in the first part of this century. The author discusses various theories of causation. No mention is made of HAPE or HACE, which had not yet been recognized (except by Ravenhill). Many excellent references. A classic report.

Schoene, R. B. Pulmonary edema at high altitude. In *Clinics in Chest Medicine*, 1986.

Schoene, R. B., et al. Effect of acetazolamide on normoxic and hypoxic exercise in humans at sea level. *Journal of Applied Physiology* 55:1772, 1983.
Acetazolamide increased ventilation and oxygenation during exercise at sea level and while breathing 12 percent oxygen, and the authors speculate that it may therefore improve performance at altitude.

————. Relationship of hypoxic ventilatory response to exercise performance on Mt. Everest. *Journal of Applied Physiology* 56:1478, 1984.

Schoene, R. B., P. H. Hackett, et al. High altitude pulmonary edema: characteristics of lung lavage fluid. *Journal of the American Medical Association* 256:63–69, 1986.

Schumacher, G., and J. Petajan. High altitude stress and retinal hemorrhages. *Archives of Environmental Health* 30:217–21, 1975.

Schwartz, J. S., H. Z. Bencowitz, et al. Air travel hypoxemia with chronic pulmonary disease. *Annals of Internal Medicine* 100:473–77, 1984.

Scoggin, C. H., T. M. Hyer, et al. High altitude pulmonary edema in the children and young adults of Leadville, Colorado. *New England Journal of Medicine* 297:1269–72, 1977; also letters in 298:914–15, 1978.

Severinghaus, J. W. Transarterial leakage: a possible mechanism for high altitude pulmonary edema. In *High Altitude Physiology: Cardiac and Respiratory Aspects,* edited by R. Porter, et al. London: Churchill Livingstone, 1971.
The author is more experienced in pulmonary patho-physiology than most other persons in this country and has a bibliography too extensive to list here.

————. Hypoxic ventilatory drive and its loss during chronic hypoxia. *Clinical Physiology* 2:57, 1972.

Shasby, D. M., S. S. Shasby, et al. Polymorphonuclear leukocyte: arachidonate edema. *Journal of Applied Physiology* 59:47–55, 1985.

Sheldon, M. I., and J. F. Green. Evidence for CO_2 chemosensitivity: effects on ventilation. *Journal of Applied Physiology* 52:1192–97, 1982.

Shields, J. L., et al. Effects of altitude acclimatization on pulmonary function in women. *Journal of Applied Physiology* 25:606–9, 1968.

Sibbald, W. J., D. R. Cunningham, et al. Non-cardiac or cardiac pulmonary edema? *Chest* 84:452–60, 1984.

Singh, I., et al. Blood coagulation changes at high altitude predisposing to pulmonary hypertension. *British Heart Journal* 34:611, 1972.

This early study of thirty-eight soldiers acclimatized to 12,000–18,000 feet for two years suggested that high-altitude pulmonary hypertension is due to occlusion of pulmonary vessels and is dependent on changes in blood coagulation.

Singh, I., and I. S. Chohan. Reversal of abnormal fibrinolytic activity, blood coagulation factors, and platelet function in high-altitude pulmonary edema with frusemide. *International Journal of Biometeorology* 17:73–81, 1973.

————. Adverse changes in fibrinolysis, blood coagulation, and platelet function in high altitude pulmonary edema and their role in its pathogenesis. *International Journal of Biometeorology* 18:33–46, 1974.

Singh, I., C. C. Kapila, et al. High altitude pulmonary edema. *Lancet,* pp. 229–34, January 30, 1965.

Singh, I., P. Khanna, et al. Acute mountain sickness. *New England Journal of Medicine* 280:175–84, 1969.

Clinical observations on 1,925 individuals with various forms of altitude illness during the Sino-Indian conflict high in the Himalayas. Relationships among the several forms of altitude illness are discussed. The largest series yet collected.

Smith, C. A., G. E. Bisgard, et al. Carotid bodies are required for acclimatization to chronic hypoxia. *Journal of Applied Physiology* 60:1003–10, 1986.

Sophocles, A. M. High altitude pulmonary edema in Vail, Colorado, 1975–82. *Western Journal of Medicine* 144:569, 1986.

Forty-seven cases of pulmonary edema, all in men, are briefly described, and the author suggests that inappropriate antidiuretic hormone action is in part responsible. The data are sketchy and there is little statistical evidence to support any of his conclusions.

Sophocles, A. M., and J. Bachman. High altitude pulmonary edema among visitors to Summit County, Colorado. *Journal of Family Practice* 17:1015–17, 1983.

Spalter, H., and G. Bruce. Ocular changes in pulmonary insufficiency. *Transactions of the American Academy of Ophthalmology and Otolaryngology,* pp. 661–76, 1964.

Staub, N. "State of the Art" Review: Pathogenesis of pulmonary edema. *American Review of Respiratory Disease* 109:358–71, 1974.
An outstanding review of all types of pulmonary edema by one of the leading authorities in respiratory physiology.

―――. The pathogenesis of pulmonary edema. *Progress in Cardiovascular Disease* 23:53–80, 1980.

Stenmark, K. R., S. L. James, et al. Leukotriene C4 and D4 in neonates with hypoxemia and pulmonary hypertension. *New England Journal of Medicine* 309:77–80, 1983.

Stewart, L. Acute pulmonary edema of high altitude. *New Zealand Medical Journal* 60:79–80, 1961.
A very early report from "down under."

Stiles, M. H. The Mexico City Olympic Games. *Minnesota Medicine* 34:9–15, 1971.

Stokes, D. C., M. E. B. Wohl, et al. Postural hypoxemia in cystic fibrosis. *Chest* 87:785–88, 1985.
Patients with cystic fibrosis are likely to have chronic hypoxia due to lung damage; this study shows that hypoxemia is worse when lying down in some individuals and may have bearing on nighttime hypoxia at altitude.

Sutton, J. R. Altitude illnesses. *Seminars in Respiratory Medicine* 5:103–215, 1983.
This issue contains a series of papers describing all aspects of altitude illness and valuable references. It is the equivalent of a small book on altitude illnesses and an excellent source.

Sutton, J. R., et al. Retinal hemorrhage at altitude. *American Alpine Journal* 22:513–18, 1980.

Sutton, J. R., C. S. Houston, et al. Effect of acetazolamide on hypoxemia during sleep at high altitude. *New England Journal of Medicine* 301:1329–31, 1979.

Sutton, J. R., and N. L. Jones. Exercise at altitude. *Annual Review of Physiology* 45:427–37, 1983.
The authors are authorities in this subspecialty, and this is an excellent background paper on altitude physiology.

Takahashi, J. S., and M. Zatz. Regulation of circadian rhythmicity. *Science* 217:1104–10, 1982.

Theodore, J., E. D. Robin, et al. Augmented ventilatory response to exercise in pulmonary hypertension. *Chest* 89:39–43, 1986.

Thomas, P. W. Rocky Mountain sickness. *Alpine Journal* 17:140 and 149, May 1894.
Brief comments reaffirming the belief that incidence of altitude sickness varies from place to place perhaps because of differences in humidity. An early summary.

Tod, M. L., and S. Cassin. Thromboxane synthase inhibition and perinatal pulmonary response to arachidonic acid. *Journal of Applied Physiology* 58:710–16, 1985.

Torre-Bueno, J. B., P. D. Wagner, et al. Diffusion limitation in normal man during exercise at sea level and at simulated altitude. *Journal of Applied Physiology* 58:989–95, 1985.

Townsley, M. I., R. J. Korthuis, et al. Effects of arachidonate on permeability and resistance distribution in canine lungs. *Journal of Applied Physiology* 58:206–10, 1985.

Veicsteinas, A., et al. Energy costs of and energy sources for alpine skiing in top athletes. *Journal of Applied Physiology* 56:1187, 1984.

Viault, F. Increase in circulating red cells. *Comptes Rendues Academy of Science,* Paris, 111:917, 1890.

Viswanathan, R., S. K. Jain, et al. Pulmonary edema of high altitude: I. Production of pulmonary edema in animals under conditions of simulated high altitude. II. Clinical, aerohemodynamic, and biochemical studies in a group with history of high altitude pulmonary edema. III. Pathogenesis. *American Review of Respiratory Disease* 100:237–349, 1977.
An extensive review of all aspects of high-altitude pulmonary edema by a distinguished Indian pathologist.

Viswanathan, R., S. Subramanian, et al. Further studies on pulmonary edema of high altitude: abnormal responses to hypoxia of men who developed high altitude pulmonary edema. *Respiration* 36:216–22, 1978.

Voelkel, N. F., M. Morganroth, et al. Potential role of arachidonic acid metabolites in hypoxic pulmonary vasoconstriction. *Chest* 89:24–26S, 1986.

Vogel, J., L. Hartley, et al. Cardiac output during exercise in altitude natives at sea level and at high altitude. *Journal of Applied Physiology* 36:173–76, 1974.

Volpe, B. T. Does chronic hypoxia cause brain injury? *Archives of Internal Medicine* 143:1866, 1983.

Wagner, P. D., G. E. Gale, et al. Pulmonary gas exchange in humans exercising at sea level and at simulated altitude. *Journal of Applied Physiology* 61:260–70, 1986.

Wagner, P. D., and J. B. West. Ventilation-perfusion relationships. In *Pulmonary Gas Exchange,* edited by J. B. West. New York: Academic Press, 1980.

Ward, M. Periodic respiration. *Annals of the Royal College of Surgeons* 52:330–34, 1973.

————. Exercise edema and mountain sickness — a field investigation. *Alpine Journal* 85:168, 1980.

Warren, S. E., J. B. Boice, et al. The athletic heart revisited: sudden death of a 28-year-old athlete. *Western Journal of Medicine* 131:441–47, 1979.

Werber, J., J. L. Ramilo, et al. Unilateral absence of a pulmonary artery. *Chest* 84:729–32, 1983.

West, J. B. State of the art: ventilation-perfusion relationships. *American Review of Respiratory Disease* 116:919–44, 1977.

————. Climbing Mount Everest without oxygen: an analysis of maximal exercise during extreme hypoxia. *Respiration Physiology* 52:265–69, 1983.

————. Do climbs to extreme altitude cause brain damage? *Lancet,* pp. 387–88, August 16, 1986.
This short communication discusses the "often heated" controversy over whether or not climbing at extreme altitude may cause lasting brain damage. The author cites (but incompletely) selected evidence pro and con, and suggests that such climbs might be discouraged because of the risk.

West, J. B., S. J. Boyer, et al. Maximal exercise at extreme altitudes on Mount Everest. *Journal of Applied Physiology* 55:688–702, 1983.

West, J. B., P. H. Hackett, et al. Pulmonary gas exchange on the summit of Mount Everest. *Journal of Applied Physiology* 55:678–87, 1983.

West, J. B., R. M. Peters, et al. Nocturnal periodic breathing at altitudes of 6,300 and 8,050 m. *Journal of Applied Physiology* 61:280–87, 1986.

Wiedman, M. Science notes: high altitude retinal hemorrhage. *American Alpine Journal* 25:113–14, 1983.

Wilkinson, Marcia. Migraine. *Encyclopedia Britannica Health Annual,* 1986.

Winslow, R. M., C. C. Monge, et al. Effect of hemodilution on O_2 transport in high altitude polycythemia. *Journal of Applied Physiology* 59:1495–1502, 1985.

Wolkove, N., et al. Effect of transcendental meditation on breathing and respiratory control. *Journal of Applied Physiology* 56:607, 1984.
During TM, the alteration in wakefulness can significantly affect the chemical and nervous control of breathing.

Woodcock, A. The search for words to describe the bad blowers. *Chest* 85:73S, Supplement, 1984.

Woodworth, J. Brief notes and bibliography of the history of mountain medicine. *Appalachia,* June 1976.
A short paper with an excellent bibliography of unusual old medical studies in the mountains.

Zimmerman, G., and R. O. Crapo. Adult respiratory distress syndrome secondary to high altitude pulmonary edema. *Western Journal of Medicine* 133:335–37, 1980.

INDEX

A-a gradient, 74–76, 217
Acapnia, 63, 133
Acclimatization, 120, 131, 201–229
  "acquired," 202
  alveoli in, 223
  drugs and, 226
  major changes in, 220
  "natural," 202
  predicting, 189, 253
  pregnancy and, 223
  recalling, 222
  red blood cells in, 182
  and accommodation, 208
Acetazolamide. See Diamox
Aconcagua, 135
Acosta, José d', 12, 13, 25, 201
Acute mountain sickness. See AMS
Adaptation, 120, 204, 223
Adenosine diphosphate. See ADP
Adenosine triphosphate. See ATP
ADH (antidiuretic hormone), 130
ADP (adenosine diphosphate),
  113–119
Aeroembolism, 156–158, 181
Aircraft, pressure in, 159, 197
Airways, description of, 70–71
Alcohol, 143, 176–177, 196
Aldrovandi, Ulisse, 39
Alexander the Great, 8, 201
Alkaline reserve, 226
Alpaca, 218
Alpine Club (London), 44
Alpine-style ascent, 179–180,
  221–222
Altitude, 254–256
  and barometric pressure, 254
  and conception, 198
  and blood pressure, 197

anemia and, 183, 204, 239
  competing at, 227
  deterioration at, 224
  limits of tolerance for, 242
  natives, 155–156, 189, 222
  training at, 226–227
Altitude illness, 122–133
  classification of, 126
  cost of, 134–135
  effect of age on, 198
  incidence of, 138
  See also AMS, CMS, HACE,
    HAPE
Alveolar gases, 80
Alveolar hypoventilation, 190–191
Alveoli, 73
Ammonium chloride as treatment,
  141
AMREE (American Medical Research Expedition to Everest),
  214–215, 218
AMS (acute mountain sickness),
  134–145
  case reports of, 10, 12, 44, 61, 125,
    135–138
  cause of, 64–65
  diet and, 142–144
  medication and, 140–142
  prevention of, 138–140
  symptoms of, 136–138
  treatment for, 141, 144
Anaerobic work, 67, 117–120
Anaxagoras, 91
Andes, 7, 135, 152–153, 207
Anemia, 183, 204, 239
Angeville, Henriette d', 231
Angioneogenesis, 219
Angiotensin, 130

Anorexia, 137
Antidiuretic hormone. *See* ADH
Archaeus, 25
Arctic Institute, 212
ARIEM (Army Research Institute of Environmental Medicine), 141, 248
Aristotle, 8, 16, 31, 85, 91
Arlandes, Marquis d', 51
Arteriosclerosis, 198
Aspirin, 141, 144, 166, 193
Ataxia, 172–175
  See also HACE
Atelectasis, 158–159
Atomic theory, 37
ATP (adenosine triphosphate), 113, 119
Auldjo, 41, 231
Auricles, 83

Bacon, Francis, 8
Baliani, Giovanni, 46
Balloons, 50–56
Balmat, Jacques, 41
Bar-headed goose, 218, 224
Barbashova, 120
Barcroft, Joseph, 64, 203–206
Barometer, history of, 18–21
Barometric pressure, 254–256
Baro-receptors, 187–188
Beaupré, Julian de, 38
Becher, J. J., 31
Beeckman, Isaac, 17
Bennett, William, 105
Benoit, Joan, 230
Bernard, Claude, 57, 95, 101, 202
Bert, Paul, 44–46, 56, 95–98
Berti, Gaspar, 24, 31, 46
Bioelectric pump, 111
Biologically active substances, 129–130, 160
Birth-control pills, 199
Bishop, Isabella, 237
Black, Joseph, 31, 50, 115
Blanchard, Jean Pierre, 54–55
Bligh, John, 153
Blindness, 192–193
Blood, 82–104
  buffer pairs, 101
  clots, 75, 183–184
  composition of, 103
  functions of, 101–104
  carrying capacity of, 95–97
  oxygen content of, 95
  pH of, 101
  platelets, 103
  pressure, control of, 84
  See also Platelets
Boerhaave, Hermann, 33

Bohr, Christian, 98
Bohr effect, 218
Borch, Ole. *See* Borrichius, Olaus
Borrichius, Olaus, 28, 31, 32
Bourrit, Marc-Theodore, 41
Boyle, Robert, 21, 24–27, 46, 89, 181
Brain
  blood flow in, 140, 171–172
  hemorrhage, 177–178
  higher centers of, 171
  impaired judgment, 124
  pressure on, 170
  See also HACE
Breathing, 66–81
  control of, 187–188
  Mayow's description of, 71
  mechanics of, 70–73
  "grunt," 76, 164
  See also Respiration
Brevoort, Meta, 237
Buchner brothers, 115
Buffer pairs, 101
Bullock-Workman, Fannie, 235–236

Campbell, Mrs., 231
Capillaries, 73, 160, 219
Carbohydrate loading, 116–117, 142–143
  See also Diet
Carbon dioxide, 32, 67, 77, 101
Carbon monoxide, 178–179, 196
  cases of poisoning, 6, 124, 196
Carbonic anhydrase (CAH), 101, 140
Cardiac catheterization, 250
Cardiac output, 217
  See also Heart
Carotid bodies, 81, 83, 188
Carotid sinus, 84, 187–188
Cavallo, Tiberias, 50
Cavendish, Henry, 32, 50–51
Cayley, George, 56
Cell, 105–111
  membrane, 110–111
  structure, 106–111
  See also Mitochondria
Cerebellum, 175
Cesalpino, Andrea, 88
Chamonix, 41, 43, 146
Charles, Jacques, 51, 54, 55
Charlière, 55
Chemo-sensitive cells, 81
Cheyne-Stokes breathing, 64, 136, 187, 251
  See also Periodic breathing
Chinese army, 211
Cho Oyu, 209
Chronic lung disease, 228

Chronic mountain sickness. *See* CMS
Cicero, 17
Cilia, 71
Circadian rhythm, 128
Circulation, 82–90
    control of, 83
    evolution of knowledge, 90
    understanding, 85
    See also Blood
Citric acid cycle, 113–116
Claude, Albert, 105
CMS (chronic mountain sickness), 125–126, 149, 191, 202
    case reports of, 189–191
Codeine, 144
Coindet, L., 204
Col du Geant, 43, 231
Colombo, Renaldo, 87
Colorado, 134, 149, 151
Commercial aircraft
    cabin pressure, 197
Competing at altitude, 227
Comrades marathon, 155
Congenital heart disease, 158–160
Consolazio, Frank, 242
Control of breathing, 187–188
    See also Respiration
Convulsions, 173
Cortés, 14
Coxwell, Henry, 56, 60
Croce-Spinelli, Joseph, 57, 59
Cymerman, Allen, 247

Da Vinci, Leonardo, 47, 62, 85
Daedalus, 47
Dalton, John, 37, 68
Dalton's law, 68
Dam-giri, 10
David-Neel, Alexandra, 237
De-acclimatization, 228
Decompression chamber, 56, 64, 163, 208, 215
    See also Operation Everest
Dehydration, 84, 143–144, 185–186
Democritus, 37
Dephlogisticated air, 34
Descartes, René, 17
Deterioration, altitude, 224
Dexamethasone, 141, 178
Diabetes, 200
Diamox, 140–141
    acclimatization and, 226
    action of, 103, 140
    preventive action of, 141–142
Diaphragm, 69

Dickinson, John, 170, 212
Diet at altitude, 142–143
    See also Carbohydrate loading
Diffusion, 73–75
    active, 109
    coefficient of, 75, 112
    facilitated, 117
    factors influencing, 70, 73
    in capillaries, 109
    See also Lungs
Digitalis, 164
Dill, Bruce, 207, 245
Dissociation curve. *See* Oxy-hemoglobin dissociation curve
Diuretics, 140–141, 164
Dive reflex, 84, 117
Diving mammals, 117
Double helix, 112–113
Douglas, C. Gordon, 205
Dragons, 9, 38–40, 47
du Faur, Freda, 237
Dutrochet, Henri, 108
Dysmetria, 176
    See also Ataxia

Earache, 181
Edema
    altitude and, 150
    exercise and, 131, 137
    sodium pump and, 117–119, 150
    See also HACE, HAPE
Egli-Sinclair, 147
Eiseman, Ben, 153
Electron microscope, 108
Empedocles, 8, 85, 91
Emphysema, 76, 190, 198
Encephalitis, 177
Engel, Claire, 233
Enzymes, 68, 116, 127–128
    definition of, 127–128
Epilepsy, 200
Erythropoietin, 217
Everest. *See* Mt. Everest
Exercise capacity, 214, 251–252
Exercise edema. *See* Edema
Exertion, 78, 143

Facilitated diffusion, 117
Farrar, J. P., 235, 236
Favre, Emmanuele, 64
Fertility, 198
Fetal hemoglobin, 100
Fetus, 199, 223
F-hemoglobin, 100
Fibrosis, pulmonary, 76
Fire air, 32, 35
Fitzgerald, Edward, 135
Fitzgerald, Mabel, 206
Fixed air, 32

Flight, 47
French Academy, 35
Frostbite, 98–99
Fulton, John, 245
Furosemide, 141, 164

Galen, 85–86
Galien, Joseph, 48
Galileo, Galilei, 17, 46, 85, 88
Gay-Lussac, Joseph Louis, 55
Genes, 112–113
Gesner, Conrad, 11, 38–40
Gilbert, Daniel, 14
Githens, John, 195
Glaisher, James, 56
Glomus cells, 188
Glycogen, 116
Graham, W. W., 241
Gray, Gary, 156–157
Graybiel, Ashton, 242
Grunt breathing, 76, 164
Guericke, Otto von, 21, 22, 27
Guglielminetti, 146
Guzmao, Lorenzo de, 48, 49

Habeler, Peter, 241
HACE (high-altitude cerebral
    edema), 169–180
  ataxia, 175
  case reports, 5, 131, 165, 169,
    173–179, 196, 238
  dexamethasone, 178
  differential diagnosis, 177–178
  disorientation, 173
  hallucinations, 173–175
  headache, 178
  mechanisms, 171–173
  prevention of, 179–180
  treatment for, 177–180
Hackett, Peter, 156, 159, 212
HAFE (high-altitude flatus expul-
    sion), 181
Haidar, Muhammad Mirza, 10, 202
Haldane, John S., 64, 109, 136, 205
Haley, Margaret, 242
Hallucinations. See HACE, HAPE
Hannibal, 8
HAPE (high-altitude pulmonary
    edema), 146–168
  age incidence, 167
  case reports, 4, 5, 64, 131, 147, 148,
    150, 151, 162, 163, 165
  cause, 160–161
  children, 167
  effect of cold air, 153
  incidence, 167
  mechanism, 153, 156–158, 160–
    161
  re-entry, 167–168

recurrent, 161, 166–167
  treatment, 162–165
Harvey, William, 88–90
Headache, 64, 136–138, 141, 178
Heart disease, 197–198
  See also Congenital heart disease,
    Pulmonary artery, absent
Heart murmurs, 200
Heart rate, 82–83
  See also Circulation
Heat loss, 73
Helmont, Johann Baptista van, 25,
    28
Hematocrit, optimal, 182
  definition, 182
Hemoglobin, 57, 67, 70, 91, 95–101
  See also Circulation, Mutant he-
    moglobins
Henderson, Yandell, 138, 205
Hermes, 127
Hertel, Horace, 243
High-altitude retinal hemorrhage,
    185–187, 212, 250
High Latitude Laboratory, 214
High permeability edema, 161
Highest permanent residents, 224
Hillary and Tensing, 209
Himalayan goose, 224
Himalayan Rescue Association,
    176
Hitchcock, Charles, 61
Hohendiuresen, 215
Holmes, Julia Archibald, 234–235
Hooke, Robert, 25–27, 94, 106
Hoppe-Seyler, Felix, 94
Hormones, 68, 127–128, 162
  definition of, 127–128
Huascaran, 236
Hultgren, Herbert, 152
Human Use Review Committee,
    249
Hurtado, Alberto, 149–150, 202
HVR (hypoxic ventilatory response),
    188–189, 221
  See also Control of respiration
Hydrogen, 51
  See also Montgolfier brothers
Hyperventilation, 77
  See also Grunt breathing
Hypothalamus, 83
Hypothermia, 38, 98–99
Hypovolemic shock, 84, 164
Hypoxic ventilatory response. See
    HVR

Ibn al-Nafis, 87
Icarus, 47
Inca, 14
Inder Singh, 211

Indian army, 167–168
Inflammable gas, 51
Inquisition, 85, 88
Insomnia, 136, 138, 212
Intermediary metabolism, 114–116
Internal environment, 105
    See also Bernard, Claude
Intermittent upper airway obstruction, 191
Interstitial edema, 158, 160, 217
    See also Edema
Intrinsic rhythm, 83
    See also Heart
Iron, 94
    deficiency, 239
Irving, R. L. G., 233
Italian research expedition, 214
IUAO, 191

Jacottet, 146–147, 150
Jarvis, Walter, 242
Jeffries, John, 54, 55
Joanne, 44
Johnson, Bev, 237
Johnson, Tom, 141
Johnson, W. H., 241
Jourdannet, Denis, 61, 204

Kidney, bleeding from, 187
    function, 102
    during acclimatization, 221
Krebs cycle, 113–116, 129

Lana-Terzi, Francesco de, 48, 62
Lasagno, Cesar, 64
Lavoisier, Antoine-Laurent, 32–35
Le Blond, Aubrey, 237
Leeuwenhoek, Anton van, 91–92
Leftward shift, 98, 218
Leullier-Ducag, 54
Leukotrienes, 129, 160–161
Liebig, Justus von, 94, 115
Livy, 8
Llama, 156, 218
Lower, Richard, 94–95

Magdeburg Spheres, 48
Maher, John, 248
Maignan, Emmanuel, 18, 19
Malpighi, Marcello, 89
Marathon runners, 142–143, 155, 230
Marco Polo, 201
Mareo, 14
    See also AMS
Margherita, Queen, 63
Maria Paradis, 231
Marsden, Kate, 237
Matthews, Brian, 73

Maximum work capacity, 209–211, 252
Mayow, John, 28–30, 56, 66, 71
McNutt, Walter, 243
Mean capillary oxygen pressure, 207
Meditation, 144
Medulla, 171
Melopeme, 230
Menghini, 94
Meningitis, 177
Menstruation, 239
Messner, Rheinhold, 241, 252
Metabolism, 112–116
Mexico, 204, 226
Meyer-Ahrens, Conrad, 61
Micro-bubbles. See Aeroembolism
Microscope, 91–92
Midbrain, 171
Migraine, 192–193
Military aircrew, 207–208
Milledge, James, 130
Mills, Bill, 214
Mitochondria, 67, 70, 77–78, 110–116, 219
Mitral valve prolapse, 200
Monge, Carlos, 189–190, 203
Monge's disease. See CMS
Mont Aiguille, 38
Mont Blanc, 41, 43, 146, 231
Mont Ventoux, 9
Monte Rosa, 63, 146
Montgolfier brothers, 50–57
Moore, Lorna, 223
Moore, Terris, 255
Morphine, 164
Morris, Carlton, 243
Mosso, Angelo, 45, 63–64, 132, 146
Mount Olympus, 7
Mt. Ararat, 7
Mt. Everest, 65, 73, 122, 209, 213, 240–241
Mt. Logan, 175, 212–213
Mt. McKinley, 214
Mt. Pilatus, 11
Mt. Washington, 196
Mouse, 20, 34, 100, 219
Mummery, Alfred, 237
Muralt, Alexander von, 202
Mutant hemoglobins, 99–101, 193–195, 218–219
    See also S-hemoglobin
Myoglobin, 67, 220

Nausea, 137
    See also AMS
Negro ancestry, 99–100
Nepal, 209
Nervous puna, 170

New pneumatic engine, 26–27
Ney Elias, 10
Nims, Leslie, 245
Nitro-aerial spirit, 28
Nitrogen bubbles, 181–182
Nitrous air, 34

O'Brien, Miriam, 236–237
Operation Everest, 242–246
Operation Everest II, 246–254
Optic nerve, 172
Oxy-hemoglobin dissociation curve,
    93–96, 218
Oxygen, 27–37, 66–81
    affinity of red cells for, 92
    benefits of, 162–164
    carrying capacity of blood, 95
    cascade, 68–70, 78, 216, 219
    content in blood, 95
    discovery of, 32–37
    gradient. *See* A-a gradient
    secretion, 109, 205–206
    transport system, 67–68, 91, 249

P-hemoglobin, 100
Paccard, François, 41
Papilledema, 172–174
Paracelsus, 25
Pariacaca, 12
Parminter sisters, 231
Partial pressure, 38, 68–69, 75–76, 78,
    251–253
Pascal, Blaise, 21–23, 31
"Passarola," 48
Pasteur, Louis, 115, 129
Patterson, John, 242
Peck, Annie, 235–236
Perier, Florin, 21–23, 31, 46
Periodic breathing, 126, 138, 187–189,
    191, 251
Peru, 149, 207
Peter of Aragon, 9
Petit, Pierre, 21
Petrarch, 9
Phantong, Mrs., 240
Pheriche, 176, 212
Phlebotomy, 182
Phlogiston, 31–35
Phospholipids, 111
Pickwickian syndrome, 190–191, 228
    See also Alveolar hypoventilation
Pikes Peak, 136, 205, 234
Pizzo, Chris, 214
Placebo effect, 141–142
Platelets, 103, 183–184
Platelet aggregates, 157–158, 161,
    166, 193
Pococke, 41
Pores in heart, 87

Porphyrins, 92
Prematurity, 198
Priestley, Joseph, 32–35, 50
Prostaglandins, 129, 166
Provera, 226
Pugh, Griffith, 209–210
Pulmonary artery
    absent, 158–160
    hypertension, 191
    pressure, 152–155, 160–161, 250
    See also HAPE
Pumps, electrolyte, 117–118
Puna, 14, 126
Puy du Dôme, 23

Quechuas, 224

Rahn, Hermann, 211
Rapmund, Garrison, 249
Ravenhill, 132, 138, 147, 170
Red blood cells, 91–94
Reeves, Jack, 140
Release hormones, 128
Renaissance, 16
Renin, 130
Rennie, Drummond, 166
Respiratory center, 81, 187–188
Respiratory exchange ratio, 142
Respiratory pigments, 92
Respiratory quotient, 142
Respiratory stimulants, 81
Rightward shift, 98, 218
Riley, Richard, 242
Roach, Robert, 165
Robert, Charles, 54
Robert, Nicholas, 54
Rock, Paul, 141
Rolaids, 141
Roskelly, John, 252
Royal Society, 26–27, 37, 92, 106
Rozier, Pilatre de, 51, 53, 55
RQ, 142
Rutherford, Daniel, 32

S-hemoglobin, 99–100, 219
    See also Sickle trait, Mutant he-
        moglobins
Salt, 143–144
Saussure, Horace-Bénédict de, 41
Scheele, Carl Wilhelm, 32–35, 66
Scheuchzer, Johann Jacob, 39, 40
Schleiden, Mathias Jakob, 108
Schneider, Edward, 205
Schoene, Robert, 156
Schwann, Theodor, 108
Scintillating scotomata, 192–193
Seals, 66
Selden, George, 242
Semicircular canals, 175

Semipermeable membranes, 73
Servetus, Michael, 85
Shearing effect, 161
Sheldon, Mary, 237
Sherpas, 214, 224
Schlagintweit brothers, 203
Shlim, David, 165
Sickle cell, 99–100
Sickle-cell crisis, 197
Sickle trait, 99–100, 193–195
Siege tactics, 221
Silver Hut expedition, 209–210
Simler, Josias, 38
Sino-Indian war, 211
Sinus pain, 181
Sivel, Theodor, 57, 124
Ski resorts, 134
Sleep
    apnea, 190–192
    breathing, 76, 78
    center, 171
    See also Periodic breathing
Sleeping pills, 195
Smith, Albert, 43
Snake River Health Service, 134
Snoring, 190–191
Sodium pump, 111, 117–119, 127, 132, 171
Soroche, 14, 126
Spaniards, 199
Speed of ascent, 166
    See also Alpine-style ascent
Spinal fluid, 171
Spiritus mundi, 31
St. Bernard, 9, 39
Stahl, Georg Ernst, 31–32
Stratton, Mary Isabella, 235
Stroke, 177, 185
Struggle responses, 120
Sujoy roy, 211
Summit, alveolar air on, 214
    condition of man on, 252–253
Surfactant, 158–159, 161
Sutton, John, 248
Swan-Ganz catheterization, 250

Tabei, Mrs., 240
Testu-Brissey, 54
Thrombophlebitis, 183
Thromboxane, 130, 160–161
Tibet, 7, 10, 224
Tidal air, 76
Torr, definition, 59

Torricelli, Evangelista, 20–21, 31, 46
Tourniquets, 164
Training, 226
Tranquilizers, 196
Transit time, 75
Transport
    active, 109–110
    facilitated, 117
    passive, 109–110
Turtle, 66, 117

V/Q mismatch, 76, 157, 159, 161
Vacuum, 17, 20–23
Vacuum pump, 22, 26, 27, 95
VanHardenbroeck, Miriam, 158
Veins, valves in, 89
Ventilation, 78
    See also Breathing, Respiration
Ventilation-perfusion mismatch. *See* V/Q mismatch
Ventricles, 83
Vesalius, Andreas, 88
Veta, 14
Vicuna, 156
Vital spirit, 17, 28, 66
Vitriol air, 32
VOMax. *See* Maximum work capacity

Walker, 56
Walker, Lucy, 235
Ward, Michael, 130
Water vapor, 69
West, John, 214–215, 224
Whales, 66
White, Paul Dudley, 152
White blood cells, 103
Whymper, Edward, 135
Wilkins, Earl, 243
Williams, Edward, 130
Winslow, Robert, 182, 218
Women, 230–241
    altitude tolerance, 239
    change in menses, 239
    iron deficiency, 239
    muscle strength, 238
    ventilation, 239
Work capacity, 209, 214
    See also Maximum work capacity

Yak, 156, 219

Zenith, 58–61, 122–123